Contents

Thyroid Cancer Guidelines Update Group   v

Notes on the development and use of the guidelines   vii

Types of evidence and grading of recommendations   ix

Abbreviations   x

Key recommendations and overview of management of thyroid cancer (differentiated and medullary)

1. Access to a multidisciplinary thyroid cancer team   xi

2. Patient focus   xi

3. Surgery   xi

4. Pathology   xi

5. Radioiodine (^{131}I) ablation therapy and external beam radiotherapy   xii

6. Aims of treatment   xii

7. Summary of management of differentiated thyroid cancer   xii

8. Follow-up of differentiated thyroid cancer   xiii

9. Medullary thyroid cancer   xiii

1   Introduction

1.1   The need for guidelines   1

1.2   Aim of the guidelines   1

1.3   Incidence   1

1.4   Prognostic factors   1

1.5   Public health and prevention   4

1.6   Screening   4

2   Presentation, diagnosis and referral

2.1   Cancer waiting times   5

2.2   Symptoms or signs that warrant investigation   6

2.3   Physical examination   6

2.4   Appropriate investigations pending hospital appointment   6

2.5   Who to refer to?   7

2.6   The role of the multidisciplinary team   7

2.7   Hospital investigations   7

2.8   Communicating the diagnosis   8

3   Fine-needle aspiration cytology

3.1   Aspiration cytology of thyroid   9

3.2   Diagnostic categories   10

4   Primary treatment of differentiated thyroid cancer

4.1   Timescale   11

4.2   Staging and risk assignment   11

4.3   Documentation   11

5   Surgery for differentiated thyroid cancer

5.1   Preparation for surgery   12

5.2   Elective surgical treatment   13

5.3   Emergency surgery   16

5.4   Surgery for locally advanced disease   16

5.5   Early post-surgical management   17

5.6   Medullary thyroid cancer   17

5.7   Surgical management of other rare malignancies of the thyroid   17

6   Radioiodine ablation and therapy for differentiated thyroid cancer

6.1   Preparation for ^{131}I ablation or therapy   18

6.2   Postoperative ^{131}I ablation   19

6.3   Diagnostic scan (^{131}I 74–150 MBq)   21

6.4   Short-term and long-term side effects of ^{131}I ablation and therapy   22

7   External beam radiotherapy

   7.1   Adjuvant external beam radiotherapy   24

   7.2   High-dose external beam radiotherapy as part of primary treatment   24

8   Post-treatment follow-up

   8.1   Voice dysfunction   25

   8.2   Management of hypocalcaemia   25

   8.3   Long-term suppression of serum thyrotrophin   26

   8.4   Role of measurement of serum thyroglobulin in long-term follow-up   26

   8.5   Role of imaging by ultrasonography and whole-body ^{131}I scanning in routine follow-up   29

9   Recurrent/persistent differentiated thyroid cancer

   9.1   Recurrence in the thyroid bed or cervical lymph nodes   30

   9.2   Metastatic disease involving lung and other soft tissue areas   30

   9.3   Bone metastases   31

   9.4   Cerebral metastases   31

   9.5   Other metastatic sites   31

   9.6   Unknown metastatic sites   31

   9.7   Palliative care   32

10   Long-term follow-up of differentiated thyroid cancer   34

11   Pregnancy and thyroid cancer

   11.1   Diagnosis of thyroid cancer in pregnancy   35

   11.2   Pregnancy in the treated patient   35

12   Thyroid cancer in childhood   37

13   Pathological reporting, grading and staging of thyroid cancers

   13.1   General principles   38

13.2   Gross description   38

13.3   Microscopic report   39

13.4   Pathological staging   39

13.5   Staging protocol   39

13.6   Grading of tumours   39

14   Management of medullary thyroid cancer

   14.1   History   41

   14.2   Hospital investigation   41

   14.3   Treatment   42

   14.4   Follow-up   44

   14.5   Pathology   44

   14.6   Molecular genetics   45

   14.7   Multiple endocrine neoplasia 2B   47

15   Registration, core dataset and audit   49

16   Thyroid cancer: a guide for general practitioners

   16.1   Raising awareness   50

   16.2   Prevention   50

   16.3   Screening   50

   16.4   Diagnosis and referral   51

   16.5   Summary of treatment of thyroid cancer   53

   16.6   Follow-up   53

Appendices

1. Assay methodology   55

2. Recognition of multiple endocrine neoplasia 2B   58

3. Search methodology   59

4. References   60

5. Patient information   70

   ▮ Patient support groups   70

   ▮ Websites with useful information for patients   70

   ▮ Leaflets for patients:
      The thyroid gland and thyroid cancer   71
      Thyroid surgery   75
      Radioactive iodine ablation and surgery   80

Thyroid Cancer Guidelines Update Group

Petros Perros (*Chair*) BSc, MBBS, MD, FRCP, Consultant Endocrinologist, Freeman Hospital, Newcastle-upon-Tyne

Susan EM Clarke MSc, FRCP, FRCR, Consultant Physician/ Senior Lecturer, Guys and St Thomas' Hospital, London

Jayne Franklyn MD, PhD, FRCP, FMedSci, Professor of Medicine, Queen Elizabeth Hospital, Birmingham

Georgina Gerrard BSc, MB, BChir, MRCP, FRCR, Consultant in Clinical Oncology, Leeds Trust

Barney Harrison MS, FRCS(Eng), FRCS(Ed), Consultant Endocrine Surgeon, Royal Hallamshire Hospital, Sheffield

Janis Hickey, Patient representative; President, British Thyroid Foundation, Harrogate

Pat Kendall-Taylor MD, DCH, FRCP, Emeritus Professor of Endocrinology, University of Newcastle, Newcastle-upon-Tyne

Anne Marie McNicol BSc, MD, MRCP(UK), FRCP(Glas), FRCPath, Reader in Pathology, University of Glasgow; Consultant Pathologist, Glasgow

Ujjal K Mallick MB, BS, MS, FRCR, Consultant Clinical Oncologist, Northern Centre for Cancer Treatment, Newcastle-upon-Tyne

Malcolm Prentice BSc, FRCP, Consultant Physician and Endocrinologist, Mayday University Hospital, Croydon

Rajesh V Thakker MD, FRCP, FRCPath, FMedSci, May Professor of Medicine, University of Oxford

John Watkinson MSc, MS, FRCS(Eng), DLO, Consultant Otolaryngologist/Head and Neck Surgeon, Queen Elizabeth Medical Centre, Birmingham

Anthony P Weetman MD, DSc, FRCP, FMedSci, Professor of Medicine and Dean of Medicine, University of Sheffield

Original (2002) Thyroid Cancer Guidelines Development Group

Pat Kendall-Taylor (*Chair*) MD, DCH, FRCP, Professor of Endocrinology, Newcastle-upon-Tyne

Geoffrey J Beckett BSc, PhD, FRCPath, Reader in Clinical Biochemistry, Edinburgh

Penny M Clark PhD, FRCPath, Consultant Clinical Scientist, Birmingham

Susan EM Clarke MSc, FRCP, Consultant Physician/Senior Lecturer, Guys and St Thomas' Hospital, London

Richard Collins FRCS(Eng), FRCS(Ed), Consultant Surgeon, Canterbury

Sharon Dobbins Chief Librarian, Sunderland Royal Hospital Trust

John Farndon BSc, MD, FRCS, Professor of Surgery, University of Bristol

Jayne Franklyn MD, PhD, FRCP, FMedSci, Professor of Medicine, Birmingham

Caroline Owen Hafiz MSc, RGN, Head and Neck Support Counsellor/Nurse, Queen Elizabeth Hospital, Birmingham

Clive Harmer FRCP, FRCR, Head of Thyroid Unit, Royal Marsden NHS Trust, London

GAW Hornett MA, FRCGP, General Practitioner, Wonersh, Guildford

Julian Kabala FRCR, Consultant Radiologist, Bristol

Julia Lawrence, Patient representative, Chipping Sodbury

Anne Marie McNicol BSc, MD, MRCP(UK), FRCP(Glas), FRCPath, Reader in Pathology, University of Glasgow; Consultant Pathologist, Glasgow

Ujjal K Mallick MB, BS, MS, FRCR, Consultant Clinical Oncologist, Newcastle-upon-Tyne

Petros Perros BSc, MBBS, MD, FRCP, Consultant Physician and Endocrinologist, Newcastle-upon-Tyne

Bruce Ponder FRS, FRCP, FMedSci, CRC Professor of Oncology, Cambridge

Malcolm Prentice BSc, FRCP, Consultant Physician and Endocrinologist, Mayday University Hospital, Croydon, Surrey

George Proud MD, FRCS, Consultant Endocrine Surgeon, Newcastle-upon-Tyne

Catharine Sturgeon BSc, PhD, Principal Clinical Scientist, Edinburgh

John Watkinson MSc, MS, FRCS(Eng), DLO, Consultant Otolaryngologist/Head and Neck Surgeon, Queen Elizabeth Medical Centre, Birmingham

Anthony P Weetman MD, DSc, FRCP, Professor of Medicine and Dean of Medicine, Sheffield

Jackie Williams, Patient representative, Ascot, Berkshire

Louiza Vini, Observer, Clinical Oncologist, Royal Marsden Hospital, London

Professional Bodies represented

British Association of Endocrine and Thyroid Surgeons

British Association of Head and Neck Oncologists

British Association of Otolaryngologists/Head and Neck Surgeons

British Association of Surgical Oncology

British Nuclear Medicine Society

British Society of Clinical Cytology

British Thyroid Association

British Thyroid Foundation

Royal College of Pathologists

Royal College of Physicians (Nuclear Medicine Committee)

Royal College of Physicians (Diabetes and Endocrinology Committee)

Royal College of Radiologists, Faculty of Clinical Oncology

Royal College of Surgeons of England

Society for Endocrinology

UK Endocrine Pathology Society

Invited Specialist Reviewers from whom comments were received on updated guidelines

Ms S Allen, Consultant Physicist, London (British Nuclear Medicine Society)

Professor N Bundred, Professor in Surgical Oncology, Manchester (British Association of Surgical Oncology)

Professor JA Fagin, Chief, Endocrinology Service, Sloan-Kettering Cancer Center, New York, USA (British Thyroid Association)

Mr A Gandhi, Consultant Breast and Endocrine Surgeon, Manchester (British Association of Endocrine and Thyroid Surgeons)

Dr TE Giles, Consultant Cytopathologist, Royal Liverpool University Hospital (British Society of Clinical Cytology)

Professor J Lazarus, Professor of Clinical Endocrinology, Cardiff (Royal College of Physicians, Diabetes and Endocrinology representative)

Dr V Lewington, Consultant Nuclear Medicine Physician, London (Royal College of Physicians and British Nuclear Medicine Society)

Dr N Reed, Consultant Clinical Oncologist, Glasgow (Faculty of Clinical Oncology, Royal College of Radiologists)

Mr N Roland, Consultant ENT/Head and Neck Surgeon, Liverpool (British Association of Head and Neck Oncologists)

Dr S Vinjamuri, Consultant in Nuclear Medicine, Liverpool (British Nuclear Medicine Society)

Notes on the development and use of the guidelines

Development of the guidelines

The first edition of *Guidelines for the management of thyroid cancer in adults* was published by the Royal College Physicians in 2002 after extensive review of the literature by representatives of professional and patient-led organisations (Royal Colleges of Physicians, Radiologists, Surgeons, Pathologists, General Practitioners, Nurses, the British Association of Endocrine Surgeons, the British Association of Otolaryngologists and Head and Neck Surgeons, the British Association of Head and Neck Oncologists, the British Nuclear Medicine Society, the Society for Endocrinology and the British Thyroid Foundation) and external refereeing.

These guidelines were updated in 2006/7 by a subgroup representing the majority of the same professional organisations in the light of recent advances in diagnosis and management of thyroid cancer. These updated guidelines place emphasis on tailoring the aggressiveness of treatment and monitoring to the individual patient and the central role of the multidisciplinary team meetings in making these decisions, based on risk assessment. In addition, the updated guidelines incorporate issues that have arisen as a result of the implementation of waiting times of the NHS Cancer Plan and the publication of *Improving outcomes in head and neck cancer* by the National Institute for Health and Clinical Excellence in 2004.[1] The second edition of the guidelines differs in emphasis on some aspects of management of thyroid cancer from recent guidelines published by the European and American Thyroid Associations. Large population follow-up data on certain areas of management of thyroid cancer are not yet available. The present document is based on a UK consensus of opinion, which the authors believe is appropriately cautious.

The updated guidelines were reviewed by several members of the original guideline group and by other external referees before publication.

The intention is that the guidelines be adopted by the individual regional cancer networks, after discussion by local clinical and managerial staff, with the addition of appropriate arrangements for use in the specific centres.

This document should be considered as a guideline only; it is not intended to serve as a standard of medical care. It should not be construed as including all the acceptable methods of care. The management plan for an individual patient must be made by the multidisciplinary team in the light of the clinical data and the diagnostic and treatment options available.

The focus of the document is the management of thyroid cancer, rather than investigation of thyroid nodules. The guideline focuses mainly on thyroid cancer in adult patients although childhood thyroid cancer is included briefly in Section 12 and in the section on medullary thyroid cancer. Guidelines on thyroid cancer in children can be found elsewhere.[2]

It is hoped that the document will provide guidance for general practitioners, general physicians, endocrinologists, surgeons, oncologists, nuclear medicine physicians, radiologists, medical physicists, biochemists and nurses, as well as those involved in managerial roles.

The guidelines are also intended to provide a basis for local and national audit and each section offers recommendations suitable for the audit process.

Funding: Development of the updated guidelines was generously supported by the British Thyroid Association.

Declaration of conflict of interests: Drs Clarke, Gerrard, Mallick and Perros have received support from Genzyme for attendance at educational meetings.

These guidelines may be photocopied or downloaded from the British Thyroid Association website:

www.british-thyroid-association.org

Types of evidence and grading of recommendations

The definition of types of evidence and the grading of recommendations used in the guidelines follow that of the Agency for Healthcare Research and Quality (formerly Agency for Health Care Policy and Research, AHCPR), as set out below:

Type of evidence

Level	Type of evidence
Ia	Evidence obtained from meta-analysis of randomised controlled trials
Ib	Evidence obtained from at least one randomised controlled trial
IIa	Evidence obtained from at least one well-designed controlled study without randomisation
IIb	Evidence obtained from at least one other type of well-designed quasi-experimental study
III	Evidence obtained from well-designed non-experimental descriptive studies, such as comparative studies, correlation studies and case-control studies
IV	Evidence obtained from expert committee reports or opinions and/or clinical experience of respected authorities

Based on AHCPR, 1992.[3]

Grading of recommendations

Grade	Evidence level	Description
A	Ia, Ib	Requires at least one randomised controlled trial as part of the body of literature of overall good quality and consistency addressing the specific recommendation
B	IIa, IIb, III	Requires availability of well-conducted clinical studies but no randomised clinical trials on the topic of recommendation
C	IV	Requires evidence from expert committee reports or opinions and/or clinical experience of respected authorities. Indicates absence of directly applicable studies of good quality

Based on AHCPR, 1994.[4]

Abbreviations

AHCPR	Agency for Health Care Policy and Research (now Agency of Healthcare Research and Quality)
AHRQ	Agency of Healthcare Research and Quality
AGES	Age at presentation, Grade of tumour, Extent, Size of primary tumour
AMES	Age at presentation, Metastases, Extent, Size of primary tumour
ARSAC	Administration of Radioactive Substances Advisory Committee (part of Health Protection Agency)
BAETS	British Association of Endocrine and Thyroid Surgeons
BAO-HNS	British Association of Otolaryngologists, Head & Neck Surgeons
CCH	C-Cell hyperplasia
CT	Computed tomography
DTC	Differentiated thyroid cancer*
EORTC	European Organisation for Research and Treatment of Cancer
FACS	Fluorescent activated cell sorter
FDG	^{18}Fluoro-deoxy-glucose
FMTC	Familial medullary thyroid cancer
FNAC	Fine-needle aspiration cytology
FTC	Follicular thyroid cancer*
GP	General practitioner
IJV	Internal jugular vein
IMRT	Intensity modulated radiotherapy
MACIS	Metastases, Age at presentation, Completeness of surgical resection, Invasion (extrathyroidal), Size

MALT	Mucosa associated lymphoid tissue
MDL	Minimum detection level
MDT	Multidisciplinary team
MEN	Multiple endocrine neoplasia
MIBG	Metaiodobenzylguanidine
MRI	Magnetic resonance imaging
MRND	Modified radical neck dissection
MTC	Medullary thyroid carcinoma*
PET	Positron emission tomography
PTC	Papillary thyroid cancer*
PTH	Parathyroid hormone
pTNM	pathologically staged according to Tumour size, Node metastases and distant Metastases
rhTSH	Recombinant human TSH
RIA	Radioimmunoassay
SAN	Spinal accessory nerve
SCM	Sternocleidomastoid muscle
T3	Triiodothyronine (liothyronine)
TFT	Thyroid function test
Tg	Thyroglobulin
TgAb	Anti-thyroglobulin antibodies
TNM	Staged according to Tumour size, Node metastases and distant Metastases
TSG	Tumour-specific group
TSH	Thyroid-stimulating hormone
WBS	Whole-body scan

*Definitions of types of thyroid cancer used in the guidelines:
Thyroid cancer: Any primary thyroid malignancy (includes differentiated thyroid cancer, medullary thyroid cancer anaplastic thyroid cancer, thyroid lymphoma and other very rare types).
Differentiated thyroid cancer: Papillary thyroid cancer and follicular thyroid cancer (includes oncocytic follicular (Hürthle) cell carcinoma).

Key recommendations and overview of management of thyroid cancer (differentiated and medullary)

These guidelines refer to the investigation and management of differentiated (papillary and follicular) and medullary thyroid cancer (MTC).

1 Access to a multidisciplinary thyroid cancer team

i   The management of differentiated thyroid cancer (DTC) (a highly curable disease) and of MTC should be the responsibility of a specialist multidisciplinary team (MDT), membership of which will normally be appointed by the regional cancer network[5] (IV, C).

ii   The timeframe for urgent referrals should comply with the Department of Health targets (section 2) (IV, C).

iii   The MDT will normally comprise surgeon, endocrinologist and oncologist (or nuclear medicine physician) with support from pathologist, medical physicist, biochemist, radiologist, specialist nurse, all with expertise and interest in the management of thyroid cancers (IV, C).

iv   Patients will normally be seen by one or more members of the MDT; a combined clinic is recommended. All members of the MDT should maintain continuing professional development (IV, C).

2 Patient focus

i   Patients should be offered full verbal and written information about their condition and their treatment (Appendix 5) (IV, C).

ii   Patients should have continuing access to a member of the MDT for guidance and support (IV, C).

3 Surgery (section 5)

The surgeon should have *training and expertise in the management of thyroid cancer* and be a member of the MDT (IV, C).

4 Pathology (section 12)

i   Pathologists dealing with thyroid tumours should have expertise and interest in thyroid cytology and histopathology (IV, C).

ii   All patients should be staged by clinical and pathological TNM staging (Tumour size, Node metastases and distant Metastases) (III, B).

iii   Patients should be assigned to the appropriate risk group (III, B). Low-risk patients are defined for the purpose of these guidelines as those in the TNM stage I, who have a probability of long-term survival greater than 98%.

5   Radioiodine (^{131}I) ablation/therapy and external beam radiotherapy (section 6)

i   An oncologist (or nuclear medicine physician) with expertise and an interest in the management of DTC should supervise this treatment and be a member of the MDT (IV, C).

ii   Those administering therapeutic ^{131}I must hold an appropriate Administration of Radioactive Substances Advisory Committee (ARSAC) certificate or must administer ^{131}I under the direction/supervision of an appropriate ARSAC certificate holder (IV, C).

iii ^{131}I ablation/therapy should be carried out only in centres with appropriate facilities (IV, C).

6   Aims of treatment

The aims of treatment are:

▪   removal of all tumour

▪   elimination of clinical, radiological or biochemical evidence of recurrence

▪   minimisation of unwanted effects of treatment.

7   Summary of management of differentiated thyroid cancer

i   All new patients should be seen by a member of the MDT, and the treatment plan should be discussed and endorsed by the MDT (section 2.5) (IV, C).

ii   Fine-needle aspiration cytology (FNAC) should be used in the planning of surgery (section 3) (III, B).

iii   Patients with a papillary thyroid cancer (PTC) more than 1 cm in diameter or with high-risk follicular thyroid cancer (FTC) should undergo near-total or total thyroidectomy. Patients with low-risk (section 1.4) FTC or PTC ≤1 cm in diameter may be treated with thyroid lobectomy alone (section 5.2) (III, B).

iv   Serum thyroglobulin (Tg) should be checked in all postoperative patients with DTC, but not sooner than six weeks after surgery (section 8.4) (IV, C).

v   Patients will normally start on triiodothyronine 20 µg tds (normal adult dosage) after the operation. This should be stopped two weeks before ^{131}I ablation or therapy (section 6.1) (IV, C).

vi   The majority of patients with a tumour more than 1 cm in diameter, who have undergone a near-total/total thyroidectomy, should have ^{131}I ablation (section 5.2) (III, B).

vii   **Always exclude pregnancy and breast feeding before administering** ^{131}I (section 6.1) (IV, C).

viii   Breastfeeding should be stopped at least four weeks and preferably eight weeks before ^{131}I ablation or therapy (section 6.1) and should not resume (IV, C).

ix   A post-ablation scan (3–10 days after ^{131}I ablation) should be performed (section 6.2) (III, B).

x   Patients treated with ^{131}I will require levothyroxine therapy in a dose sufficient to suppress the serum thyroid-stimulating hormone (TSH) to <0.1 mIU/L (III, B). Levothyroxine can be commenced three days after ^{131}I in a dose sufficient to suppress TSH to <0.1 mIU/L. In patients confirmed to be low risk, a serum TSH <0.5 mIU/L is probably acceptable (section 8.3).

xi   Reassessment with a whole-body scan (WBS) after stopping levothyroxine for four weeks, and stimulated serum Tg is indicated no earlier than six months after ^{131}I ablation. If abnormal uptake of the tracer is detectable, a ^{131}I therapy dose should be given and a post-treatment scan (3–10 days after ^{131}I therapy) performed. Following this, the patient should restart levothyroxine (sections 8.4 and 8.5) (III, B).

xii   In low-risk (section 1.4) patients, measurement of Tg after TSH stimulation alone (ie without a diagnostic ^{131}I WBS) may be adequate. In such cases ultrasonography of the neck 6–12 months after thyroidectomy is indicated (section 8.5) (III, B).

xiii   If there is suspicion of residual disease, further scans should be carried out, usually six months after ^{131}I therapy (IV, C).

xiv   External beam radiotherapy is only occasionally used, for patients with pT4 tumours (TNM staging) and presumed residual disease in the neck which is not amenable to further surgery, particularly when the tumour does not take up ^{131}I (section 7). External beam radiotherapy also has a role as a palliative measure in patients with advanced local or distant disease (section 9).

8   Follow-up of differentiated thyroid cancer

Follow-up should be lifelong (IIb, B) for the following reasons:

- The disease has a long natural history.
- Late recurrences are not rare and can be treated successfully.
- Regular follow-up is also necessary for monitoring of treatment (TSH suppression, the consequences of supraphysiological levothyroxine replacement, treatment of hypocalcaemia).
- **Lifelong suppression** of serum TSH level below normal (<0.1 mIU/L) is one of the main components of treatment in high-risk cases (III, B).
- Patients should be monitored for late side effects of ^{131}I treatment (IV, C).

Surveillance for recurrence of disease is essential and is based on:

- annual clinical examination (IV, C)
- annual measurement of serum Tg and TSH (IV, C)
- diagnostic imaging and FNAC when indicated (III, B).

Support and counselling are necessary, particularly in relation to pregnancy (IV, C).

9   Medullary thyroid cancer (section 14)

i   The initial evaluation of suspected MTC includes FNAC and measurement of plasma calcitonin (III, B).

ii   The MDT should include or have access to a clinical genetics service and *RET* gene testing (IV, C).

iii   All patients with MTC should be offered genetic counselling and *RET* mutation analysis, whether or not there is an evident family history (**IV, C**).

iv   *RET* mutation testing should include exons 10, 11, 13, 14, 15 and 16; screening of exons 10 and 11 alone is an incomplete test (**III, B**).

v   Familial MTC (FMTC) represents 25% of all cases of MTC and associated endocrinopathies should be sought (MEN2A and 2B) (**IV, C**).

vi   Phaeochromocytoma and primary hyperparathyroidism should be excluded in new patients with MTC by measuring 24-hour urine catecholamines and metanephrines and serum calcium (**IV, C**).

vii   The minimum treatment is total thyroidectomy and level VI node dissection (**III, B**).

viii   Prophylactic surgery should be considered in disease-free carriers of germ line *RET* mutations. Surgery should be performed in MEN2A patients before the age of 5 years (**III, B**). MTC occurs early in MEN2B and is particularly aggressive; thyroid surgery should be performed ideally by the age of 12 months. In children from FMTC kindred, surgery should be postponed until after 10 years of age (**III, B**).

ix   Lifelong follow-up is essential and includes monitoring of the tumour marker calcitonin (**III, B**).

1 Introduction

1.1 The need for guidelines

In spite of advances in diagnostic methods, surgical techniques and clinical care, there are differences in survival of patients with thyroid cancer in different countries, and the outcome in the UK prior to 1989 appeared to be worse than in other western European nations.[6] The reasons for this are unclear and may be multifactorial. It is hoped that the establishment of national guidelines for thyroid cancer, and their implementation through local protocols, would lead to better care and subsequent improvement in survival for patients with thyroid cancer in the UK.

1.2 Aim of the guidelines

The intention is to provide guidance for all those involved in the management of patients with differentiated thyroid cancer (DTC). This document is not intended as a guideline for the investigation of thyroid nodules.

A summary of the key recommendations for the management of adult differentiated and medullary thyroid cancer (MTC) is provided (see previous section). Randomised trials are often not available in this setting. Therefore, evidence is based on large retrospective studies and the level of evidence according to the Agency for Healthcare Research and Quality (AHRQ)[3,4] is largely II–IV.

The three main aims of the guidelines are:
- to improve the long-term overall and disease-free survival of patients with thyroid cancer
- to enhance the health-related quality of life of patients with thyroid cancer
- to improve the referral pattern and management of patients with thyroid cancer.

1.3 Incidence

The incidence of thyroid cancer appears to be increasing slowly. In the period 1971–95, the annual UK incidence was reported at 2.3 per 100,000 women and 0.9 per 100,000 men, with approximately 900 new cases and 250 deaths recorded in England and Wales due to thyroid cancer every year.[7] In 2001, data from Cancer Research UK showed 1,200 new cases in England and Wales, with a reported annual incidence for the UK of 3.5 per 100,000 women and 1.3 per 100,000 men.[8] Thyroid cancer is the most common malignant endocrine tumour, but represents only about 1% of all malignancies.[7]

1.4 Prognostic factors

The long-term outcome of patients treated effectively for DTC is usually favourable. The overall 10-year survival rate for middle-aged adults with DTC is 80–90%. However, 5–20% of patients develop local or regional recurrences and 10–15% distant metastases. Nine per cent of patients with a diagnosis of thyroid cancer die of their disease.[9]

It is important to assess risk in patients with DTC using a prognostic scoring system: this enables a more accurate prognosis to be given and the appropriate treatment decisions to be made. The following staging methodologies are used:

TNM	Tumour size, Node metastases and distant Metastases
AMES	Age at presentation, Metastases, Extent, Size of primary tumour
MACIS	Metastases, Age at presentation, Completeness of surgical resection, Invasion (extrathyroidal), Size
EORTC	European Organisation for Research and Treatment of Cancer methodology
AGES	Age at presentation, Grade of tumour, Extent, Size of primary tumour

Any of them can be used to assign patients to the high-risk or low-risk band, based on well-established prognostic factors (detailed below), but TNM and MACIS probably yield the most useful prognostic information.[10,11]

Low-risk patients are defined for the purpose of these guidelines as those classified by the 5th edition of the TNM[10,12] as stage I category, who have a probability of long-term survival greater than 98%.

The principal factors contributing to *high risk* are older age, male gender, poorly differentiated histological features, tumour size, extrathyroidal invasion and metastatic spread. Treatment also influences prognosis.[13]

Age

Age at the time of diagnosis is one of the most consistent prognostic factors in patients with papillary and follicular thyroid cancer (FTC). The risk of recurrence and death increases with age, particularly after the age of 40 years.[13–18] Young children, under the age of 10 years, are at higher risk of recurrence than older children or adolescents.[19,20]

Gender

The male gender has been reported as an independent risk factor in some but not all studies.[9,16,17,21]

Histology

The prognosis of papillary thyroid cancer (PTC) is better than that of follicular thyroid cancer (FTC). However, if the confounding effects of age and extent of tumour at diagnosis are removed, survival rates are comparable.[13,16,22–24] Within the PTC group, poorer prognosis is associated with specific histological types[25–28] and the degree of cellular differentiation and vascular invasion.[14,29] 'Widely invasive' and 'vascular invasion' are features of follicular cancers associated with a poorer prognosis.[28,30] Poorly differentiated follicular cancers (insular carcinoma) and oncocytic follicular (Hürthle) cell carcinomas are also associated with a poorer outcome.[16,17,31]

Tumour extent

The risk of recurrence and mortality correlates with the size of the primary tumour.[13,15–18,21,31] Extrathyroidal invasion,[13,15–18,29,32,33] lymph node metastases,[13,16,17,31] and distant metastases[32,34–36] are all important prognostic factors.

Prognostic scoring systems for differentiated thyroid cancer

Staging

The 5th edition of the TNM classification is recommended[10,12,12a,12b] (III, B). The MACIS scoring system is also useful in assessing risk.[29]

Table 1. The TNM system.
(a) Classification according to tumour, nodes and metastases

Primary tumour

pT1   Intrathyroidal tumour, ≤1 cm in greatest dimension

pT2   Intrathyroidal tumour, >1-4 cm in greatest dimension

PT3   Intrathyroidal tumour, >4 cm in greatest dimension

pT4   Tumour of any size, extending beyond thyroid capsule

pTX   Primary tumour cannot be assessed

Regional lymph nodes (cervical or upper mediastinal)

N0   No nodes involved

N1   Regional nodes involved
If possible, subdivide
N1a Ipsilateral cervical nodes
N1b Bilateral, midline or contralateral cervical nodes or mediastinal nodes

NX   Nodes cannot be assessed

Distant metastases

M0   No distant metastases

M1   Distant metastases

MX   Distant metastases cannot be assessed

(b) Papillary or follicular carcinoma staging

	Under 45 years	45 years and older
Stage I	Any T, any N, M0	pT1, N0, M0
Stage II	Any T, any N, M1	pT2, N0, M0
		pT3, N0, M0
Stage III		pT4, N0, M0
		Any pT, N1, M0
Stage IV		Any pT, any N, M1

Undifferentiated or anaplastic carcinomas: **All are Stage IV.**

(c) 10-year mortality rates for differentiated (papillary or follicular) thyroid cancer.[10]

Stage	10-year cancer-specific mortality (%)
I	1.7
II	15.8
III	30
IV	60.9

1.5 Public health and prevention

Nuclear fallout is a well recognised cause of an increase in the risk of thyroid cancer in children. Following the Chernobyl accident, the incidence of thyroid cancer rose several hundred times in children in the region.

Therapeutic and diagnostic X-rays in childhood are also possible causes of thyroid cancer in adults; exposure to these sources should be limited whenever possible.

In cases of populations or individuals being contaminated with ^{131}I, the thyroid can be protected by administering potassium iodide.[36a,37,38]

1.6 Screening

At present there is no screening programme to detect thyroid cancer for the general population.

Screening is possible for familial MTCs associated with specific oncogene mutations.

The genetic basis of papillary, follicular and anaplastic thyroid cancer has been investigated and the roles and potential prognostic value of several genes, eg *RET, TRK, ras, BRAF* and *p53*, have been identified. Testing for these genes is not routinely available in clinical practice.[39]

The following are considered to be risk factors for thyroid cancer:[20,40–48]

- history of neck irradiation in childhood
- endemic goitre
- Hashimoto's thyroiditis (risk of lymphoma)
- family or personal history of thyroid adenoma
- Cowden's syndrome (macrocephaly, mild learning difficulties, carpet-pile tongue, with benign or malignant breast disease)
- familial adenomatous polyposis
- familial thyroid cancer.

While screening generally is not possible, a family history for thyroid cancer should be taken in each case and if there is a strong familial incidence of thyroid cancer or association with other cancers, genetic advice should be considered in appropriate cases from the regional genetics service (**IV, C**).

2 Presentation, diagnosis and referral

Thyroid nodules are common in adults and may be detected by palpation in 10% of women and 2% of men.[49] The prevalence may be as high as 50% or more if sensitive imaging such as ultrasonography is used. The vast majority of thyroid nodules are benign and do not require urgent referral. Furthermore, thyroid cancer is uncommon in patients who are not euthyroid, and assessment of biochemical thyroid status is useful in deciding on the referral pathway by the general practitioner (GP). (See also section 16, A guide for GPs.)

2.1 Cancer waiting times

Referrals for suspected cancer are required to be seen in secondary care within 2 weeks, as set out in the Department of Health Cancer Plan document, *Cancer waiting targets: a guide.*[50] Specialists in secondary care have a maximum of 31 days from 'decision to treat' to first definitive treatment and a maximum of 62 days from urgent GP referral for suspected cancer to first definitive treatment (Fig 1).

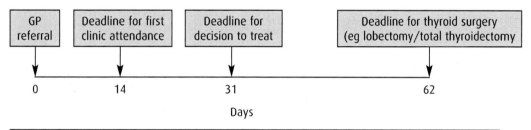

Fig 1. Thyroid cancer waiting times.

In the case of thyroid nodules, the time of 'decision to treat' is when a decision to proceed to thyroidectomy is made after discussion with the patient (section 3.1). Decisions to treat thyroid cancers should follow multidisciplinary team (MDT) discussions (**IV, C**). The date of first definitive treatment is the date of thyroidectomy (either lobectomy or total thyroidectomy).

The most common presentation of thyroid cancer is a newly discovered palpable thyroid nodule or increase in size of a pre-existing nodule. However, the vast majority of patients (95%) presenting in this manner have benign disease. Furthermore the prognosis of those who harbour a malignancy is generally excellent. **The Thyroid Cancer Guidelines Update Group recommends that thyroid nodules need not be referred under the 2-week cancer rule unless there are suspicious clinical features (section 2.2), and that optimum care can be delivered by adopting a target of 4 weeks from referral to first assessment in secondary care for all other thyroid modules (IV, C).**

Hospitals providing secondary care for patients with suspected thyroid cancer should develop well defined and streamlined pathways of referral and care (**IV, C**). Designated diagnostic clinics with appropriate resources for patients with thyroid lumps are desirable.

2.2 Symptoms or signs that warrant investigation

Thyroid nodules and goitre are common and often noted coincidentally when patients are being imaged for other reasons. The vast majority (95%) of cases have benign disease. GPs must exercise common sense in selecting which cases should be referred and with what degree of urgency.

Patients with thyroid nodules who may be managed in primary care (**IV, C**):

- Patients with a history of a nodule or goitre which has not changed for years and who have no other worrying features (ie adult patient, no history of neck irradiation, no family history of thyroid cancer, no palpable cervical lymphadenopathy).
- Patients with a non-palpable asymptomatic nodule <1 cm in diameter discovered coincidentally by imaging of the neck without other worrying features.

Patients who should be referred non-urgently (**IV, C**):

- Patients with nodules who have abnormal thyroid function tests (TFTs). These patients should be referred to an endocrinologist; thyroid cancer is very rare in this group.
- Patients with a history of sudden onset of pain in a thyroid lump (likely to have bled into a benign thyroid cyst).
- Patients with a thyroid lump which is newly presenting or increasing in size over months.

Symptoms needing urgent referral (2-week rule)[50] (**IV, C**):

- Unexplained hoarseness or voice changes associated with a goitre.
- Thyroid nodule in a child.
- Cervical lymphadenopathy associated with a thyroid lump (usually deep cervical or supraclavicular region).
- A rapidly enlarging painless thyroid mass over a period of weeks (a rare presentation of thyroid cancer and usually associated with anaplastic thyroid cancer or thyroid lymphoma).

Symptoms needing immediate (same day) referral (**IV, C**):

- *Stridor* associated with a thyroid lump.

2.3 Physical examination

The patient should have a full examination focusing on inspection and palpation of the neck, including the region of the thyroid, the deep cervical nodes and all other node groups in the neck, particularly the supraclavicular nodes. The pulse and blood pressure should be recorded (**IV, C**).

2.4 Appropriate investigations pending hospital appointment

i   TFTs should be requested by the GP (**IV, C**).

ii Euthyroid patients with a thyroid nodule may have thyroid cancer and should be referred to a member of a multidisciplinary thyroid cancer team (section 2.4) (**IV, C**).

iii Patients with hyper- or hypothyroidism and a nodular goitre without suspicious features should be referred routinely to an endocrinologist (**IV, C**).

iv Initiation of other investigations by the GP, such as ultrasonography or isotope scanning, is likely to result in unnecessary delay in making the diagnosis of cancer[52] and is not recommended (IIb, B).

2.5 Who to refer to?

i   Patients should be referred to a surgeon, endocrinologist, clinical oncologist or nuclear medicine physician who has a specialist interest in thyroid cancer and is a member of the MDT (see Key Recommendation 1)[1] (IV, C).

ii The local cancer centre or cancer unit[5] should provide clear guidance to GPs on referral pathways to secondary care (IV, C).

2.6 The role of the multidisciplinary team

All patients with DTC should be seen within an MDT framework as required by the NHS Cancer Services Standards.[1,51]

i   Patients with suspected thyroid cancer will usually be seen initially by an individual member of the MDT, who will be working according to guidelines (IV, C).

ii Clinicians may proceed with the diagnostic work-up of patients with suspected thyroid cancer without necessarily involving the MDT at every step until a diagnosis is reached or a therapeutic procedure is being considered (IV, C).

iii The treatment plan and care of each newly diagnosed patient should be discussed and supervised by a core team (physician and surgeon) in consultation with other members of the MDT. This discussion should be recorded in the patient's notes (IV, C).

iv Close communication between members of the MDT is key for delivering optimal care and a combined clinic is the preferred format.

v   The management of MTC is best delivered by a dedicated group of clinicians within the MDT who have special expertise in this complex disease (IV, C).

2.7 Hospital investigations

Essential assessments

i   Review of TFTs[52] (IIb, B).

ii Fine-needle aspiration cytology (FNAC) with or without ultrasound guidance[53,54] (IIb, B). Ultrasound is helpful in reducing the number of inadequate fine-needle aspirates.[54a]

iii Note that the measurement of serum thyroglobulin (Tg) before thyroidectomy has no diagnostic or prognostic value and should not be undertaken[55] (III, B).

Other assessments

A number of other investigations may be undertaken, but these are not routinely indicated.

i   Thyroid autoantibodies may be measured if there is a suspicion of concurrent autoimmune thyroid disease (lymphoma of the thyroid occurs almost exclusively on a background of Hashimoto's thyroiditis).

ii Magnetic resonance imaging (MRI) or computed tomography (CT) scanning is indicated when the limits of the goitre cannot be determined clinically or for fixed tumours or in patients with haemoptysis. It is important to avoid the use of iodinated contrast media when undertaking CT scans as these may reduce the subsequent radioiodine uptake by thyroid tissue. Gadolinium-enhanced MRI may provide useful information without compromising subsequent radioiodine uptake by any remaining thyroid tissue. Ultrasound scanning is rarely diagnostic, but may be of value in aiding FNAC and in the evaluation of coexisting non-dominant nodules or cervical lymphadenopathy.[54]

iii Basal plasma calcitonin levels may be useful if MTC is suspected[56,57] but is not recommended routinely for all thyroid nodules (IV, C).

iv Flow-volume loop studies may be indicated if upper airways obstruction is suspected.[58]

v Radioisotope studies are usually non-diagnostic of thyroid cancer and therefore of limited value particularly in iodine-replete countries.[59,60]

vi Excisional biopsy is rarely indicated and when tissue diagnosis prior to intervention is difficult to obtain by FNAC, and would alter patient management (typically when lymphoma is suspected), core biopsy with or without ultrasound guidance is recommended (IV, C).

2.8 Communicating the diagnosis

Informing the primary care team

i The GP should be informed (by telephone or fax) within 24 hours[51] of the diagnosis of cancer being communicated to the patient for the first time, and should be made aware of the information which has been given to the patient and of the planned treatment (IV, C).

ii Subsequently any alterations in prognosis, management or drug treatment should be communicated promptly (IV, C).

Informing the patient

i The patient should be informed of the diagnosis of cancer by a member of the MDT; facilities should be available for this to be done during a private, uninterrupted consultation (IV, C).

ii A trained nurse specialist should be available to provide additional counselling if required (IV, C).

iii Whenever possible a relative or friend should attend the consultation and accompany the patient home (IV, C).

iv Written information concerning thyroid cancer and its treatment and possible complications should be available to the patient (Appendix 5) (IV, C).

v A prognosis should not be offered before adequate staging information is available (IV, C).

vi Patients may have difficulty assimilating all this information at a single consultation and an opportunity for further explanation/discussion should be offered (IV, C).

3 Fine-needle aspiration cytology

3.1 Aspiration cytology of thyroid

The clinical usefulness of FNAC depends on obtaining adequate material for diagnosis, which requires close co-operation between biomedical scientists, pathologists and clinicians managing the patients so that appropriate procedures are set up, carried out and monitored.

i   FNAC should be used in the planning of surgery[60–62] (III, B). The diagnosis of thyroid malignancy cannot always be made by FNAC alone. In many cases an operative procedure will be required to establish a diagnosis of malignancy. Ideally, procedures should be in place to allow adequacy of the sample to be assessed at the time of aspiration and for material to be retained for ancillary tests if necessary.

ii   Thyroid cytology should be reported by a cytopathologist with a special interest in thyroid disease who should be a member of the MDT. There should be a correlation between the cytological diagnosis and any subsequent histology (IV, C).

iii   Aspiration may be performed by a cytopathologist, endocrinologist, surgeon, nuclear medicine physician, oncologist or radiologist with expertise and interest in thyroid disease. However, they should be trained in good practice, should perform sufficient aspirates to maintain expertise and their performance should be monitored (IV, C). FNAC can readily be carried out without ultrasound guidance if the lesion is palpable. In many centres there is a move towards the use of ultrasound guidance as this increases confidence that the lesion has been appropriately sampled. Care must be taken to avoid contamination of the samples with ultrasound gel when it is used.

iv   All FNAC requests should include full clinical details and details of the aspiration procedure, including the site of the abnormality and the site of sampling (IV, C).

v   Where cysts are aspirated the pathologist should be informed as to whether or not there was complete resolution of the mass after aspiration. All the material aspirated (not just a sample) should be sent to the laboratory without fixation (and therefore without delay) as tumours may present as cysts (IV, C). Any residual mass should be immediately re-aspirated and the specimens identified separately (IV, C). Cysts can be reported along the lines outlined below, but the stipulation regarding adequacy can be relaxed where a cyst aspirate has resulted in resolution of the mass.

vi   The descriptive report will inform the clinical decisions on management, but many centres find it useful to add a numerical coding, such as that defined below (section 3.2). This helps both in guiding discussion on further management and in audit.

vii In some instances, particularly for the diagnosis of malignancy, ancillary tests are required to complete the cytological diagnosis. This requires appropriate material to be retained at the time of the FNAC and is facilitated by the attendance of laboratory staff at the procedure. Immediate assessment of the cytology sample allows a decision whether immunocytochemistry, molecular analysis or flow cytometry is required. Liquid-based cytology is used in some laboratories but does not allow for either immediate assessment or flow cytometry and is not the preferred method for immunocytochemistry in all centres. Liquid-based cytology may be a useful adjunct to direct smears. Where appropriate, the results of additional investigations should be included in the text of the report, eg immunopositivity for calcitonin in medullary carcinoma; immunocytochemistry, fluorescence-activated cell sorting (FACS) analysis or molecular analysis of light chain (κ or λ) restriction in lymphoma (IV, C).

viii FNAC can also be used in the diagnosis of suspicious lymph nodes (with the same requirements for assessing adequacy as for thyroid).

ix All cases with suspected or definitive diagnosis of neoplasia, or in whom there are discrepancies between clinical or radiological findings and cytology diagnosis, should be discussed at the MDT meeting (IV, C).

3.2 Diagnostic categories

As noted above (section 3.1vi), diagnostic categories should be used alongside the final cytology assessment only after a text report.

Thy1	Non-diagnostic (inadequate or where technical artefact precludes interpretation; adequate smears usually contain six or more groups of over 10 thyroid follicular cells, but the balance between cellularity and colloid is more important).
Action	FNAC should be repeated. Ultrasound guidance may permit more targeted sampling where the initial FNAC has been undertaken by palpation. Cysts containing colloid or histiocytes only, in the absence of epithelial cells, should be classified as Thy1 but should be clearly described as cysts. If the cyst has been aspirated to dryness with no residual mass, clinical/ultrasound follow-up alone may be sufficient.
Thy2	Non-neoplastic (with the descriptive report documenting the features consistent with a colloid nodule or thyroiditis). Cysts may be classified as Thy2 if benign epithelial cells are present.
Action	Two non-neoplastic results 3–6 months apart are generally advisable to exclude neoplasia.[61,62] However, there are frequent cases where a reliable multidisciplinary benign diagnosis can be achieved with a single well targeted aspirate. In high clinical risk group cases, the decision to proceed to lobectomy may be made even with a benign FNAC diagnosis.
Thy3	(i) Follicular lesion/suspected follicular neoplasm. While some of these will be tumours, many will be shown to be hyperplastic nodules on surgical excision. The descriptive text will indicate the level of suspicion of neoplasia.
Action	Most of these patients should be treated by surgical removal of the lobe containing the nodule[61,62] (III, B). These cases should be discussed in the MDT meeting if a therapeutic procedure is being considered (IV, C). Completion thyroidectomy may be necessary if the histology proves malignant. In some cases (based on clinical or radiological features) it will be more appropriate to see whether this decision is supported by the MDT.
Thy3	(ii) There may be a very small number of other cases where the cytological findings warrant inclusion in this category rather than Thy2 or Thy4 (eg worrying features but cells too scanty to qualify for Thy4, repeat FNAC advised). The text of the report should indicate the worrying findings (IV, C).
Action	These cases should be discussed in the MDT to decide on the appropriate course of action (IV, C).
Thy4	Suspicious of malignancy (suspicious, but not diagnostic, of papillary, medullary or anaplastic carcinoma, or lymphoma).
Action	Surgical intervention is usually indicated for suspected cancer[61,62] (IIb, B). All these cases should be discussed by the MDT (IV, C). Where Thy4 assessment has been given because of the absence of material for immunocytochemistry (medullary carcinoma) or flow cytometry (lymphoma), the aspirate should be repeated.
Thy5	Diagnostic of malignancy (unequivocal features of papillary, medullary or anaplastic carcinoma, lymphoma or metastatic tumour).
Action	The diagnosis should be discussed at the MDT meeting where further management should be agreed (IV, C). Surgical intervention is indicated for DTC and MTC[61,62] (IIb, B), depending on tumour size, clinical stage and other risk factors. Appropriate further investigation, radiotherapy and/or chemotherapy is indicated for anaplastic thyroid carcinoma, lymphoma or metastatic tumour.

4 Primary treatment of differentiated thyroid cancer

4.1 Timescale

i Patients with suspected thyroid cancer should normally be seen within *2 weeks* (section 2) (**IV, C**).

ii If there are progressive/severe respiratory problems associated with a thyroid mass, patients must be referred and seen without delay (**IV, C**).

iii Patients with new onset of stridor and a thyroid mass must be assessed as emergency cases (**IV, C**).

iv Decisions should be made promptly with respect to diagnosis and treatment (maximum 31 days from diagnosis to first treatment and 62 days from urgent referral to first treatment (section 2, Fig 1)) (**IV, C**).

v ^{131}I ablation should be offered within 3–8 weeks after surgery[13] (**IV, C**).

4.2 Staging and risk assignment

i Patients should be staged using the TNM classification (section 1.4), and assigned to the appropriate risk group (section 1.4) (**III, B**).

ii Low-risk patients are defined in section 1.4.

4.3 Documentation

The following should be recorded in the notes (**IV, C**):

- family history
- date of surgery
- name of surgeon, assistant and anaesthetist
- extent of surgery
- complications of surgery
- presence or absence of metastases including number and location of lymph nodes
- FNAC, histology and pathologically staged according to TNM (pTNM) staging
- curative or palliative intent
- date of ^{131}I ablation/therapy
- dose of ^{131}I ablation/therapy and side effects
- follow-up arrangements.

5 Surgery for differentiated thyroid cancer

The relationship between volume of thyroid surgery by individual surgeons and outcome is complex.[63,64] However, there is a strong case for patients with thyroid cancer to be operated on and treated by clinicians who have appropriate training and experience.

The MDT will consult with the relevant national bodies (such as the British Association of Endocrine and Thyroid Surgeons (BAETS), the British Association of Otolaryngologists, Head & Neck Surgeons (BAO-HNS), specialist groups of the Royal Colleges, and the tumour-specific group (TSG) of the regional cancer network) to decide who are to be the surgical and non-surgical specialists involved in the management of thyroid cancer (IV, C).

A number of compliance measures recommended by the *Manual of cancer services standards*[5] relate to thyroid cancer surgery and include a named surgeon to perform lymph node resection and complex surgical procedures to be performed in the same hospital of the MDT.[65]

Regular audit of outcomes and complications of surgery undertaken by the MDT will help clinicians to maintain their skill and professional development.

5.1 Preparation for surgery

i   A hospital providing therapeutic surgery for patients with thyroid cancer should have a nominated surgeon who will be a member of the MDT with specific training in and experience of thyroid oncology[1] (IV, C). Membership of the BAETS mandates annual returns and provides comparative performance data on surgical numbers and outcome measures.

ii   Informed consent should be obtained from all patients after full discussion; the operating surgeon should normally obtain the consent (IV, C).

iii The specific complications of thyroid surgery should be discussed as well as those complications which can occur in any surgical procedure; this should be recorded in the notes. Patients should be provided with information sheets (Appendix 5) (IV, C).

iv   Prophylactic heparin preparations are not required for routine use in patients undergoing thyroid surgery (IV, C). Thromboembolism prophylaxis should be used in all cases in the form of graduated compression hose (thromboembolism deterrent stockings) and peri-operative calf compression devices[65,65a] (Ia, A).

v   In patients with suspected or proven thyroid cancer, assessment of vocal cord function is strongly recommended prior to surgery[66] (IV, C).

vi   Pre-operative cross-sectional imaging with CT (without contrast) or MRI may be indicated if there is bulky disease or vocal cord paralysis.[66]

vii Ultrasonography of the neck before thyroid surgery may be valuable in planning surgery, depending on the individual surgeon's preference and availability of ultrasonographic expertise.[67]

5.2   Elective surgical treatment

Thyroid surgery

The mainstay of treatment for DTC is surgery.[9,13,68–70] Compliance with appropriate and clear definitions of surgical procedures is essential. A diagnostic thyroid FNAC (Thy5) enables treatment to be planned and discussed with the patient prior to surgery.[71–73]

i   The following terms should be used (IV, C):

- *Lobectomy:* the complete removal of one thyroid lobe including the isthmus.
- *Near-total lobectomy:* a total lobectomy leaving behind only the smallest amount of thyroid tissue (significantly less than 1 g) to protect the recurrent laryngeal nerves.
- *Near-total thyroidectomy:* the complete removal of one thyroid lobe (lobectomy) with a near-total lobectomy on the contralateral side *or* a bilateral near-total procedure. This should be clearly defined in the operation note.
- *Total thyroidectomy:* the removal of both thyroid lobes, isthmus and pyramidal lobe.

The terms 'subtotal lobectomy' and 'subtotal thyroidectomy' are imprecise and should be avoided. The classically described subtotal lobectomy or subtotal thyroidectomy procedures are inappropriate for the treatment of thyroid cancer. If a total thyroidectomy is not carried out, the surgeon should document the exact extent of surgery to each lobe (IV, C).

ii   The recurrent laryngeal nerve/s should be identified and preserved in virtually all instances (IV, C). Permanent damage to a recurrent laryngeal nerve should occur in significantly less than 5% of patients who have undergone surgery for thyroid cancer. Bilateral injuries are extremely rare. Nerve injury rates are higher after re-operative surgery.[71]

iii   Infiltration by tumour contributes to recurrent laryngeal nerve palsy rates in malignant disease. In *benign disease* and in small thyroid cancers (ie in the absence of recurrent laryngeal nerve infiltration) total thyroidectomy is associated with no higher risk of nerve injury than in lesser procedures, provided the nerves are identified.[74]

iv   Attempts should be made to preserve the external branch of the superior laryngeal nerves by ligation of the superior thyroid vessels at the capsule of the gland (IV, C). External laryngeal nerve injury has an associated morbidity, particularly in voice-quality changes. Injury rates may be higher than for recurrent laryngeal nerve damage.[75,76]

v   Parathyroid glands should whenever possible be identified and preserved (IV, C). If their vascular supply is compromised, the gland/s should be excised and reimplanted into muscle[77](III, B). Lymph node dissection in the central compartment (level VI) is associated with an increased risk of postoperative hypoparathyroidism.[78,79]

Lymph node surgery

The terms listed below for lymph node groups and surgery should be used (IV, C).

Lateral compartment of neck

Level I   Submental and submandibular nodes.

Level II   Deep cervical chain nodes from the skull base to the level of the hyoid, which are further divided by their relationship to the accessory nerve: IIa (medial) and IIb (lateral).

Level III   Deep cervical chain nodes from the level of the hyoid to the level of the cricoid.

Level IV   Deep cervical chain nodes from the level of the cricoid to the suprasternal notch.

Level V   Posterior triangle nodes, which can be divided by their relationship to the omohyoid muscle into Va (above) and Vb (below).

Central compartment of neck

Level VI   Pretracheal and paratracheal nodes from the hyoid bone superiorly to the level of the sternal notch inferiorly and to the carotid arteries laterally.

Mediastinal nodes

Level VII   Superior mediastinal nodes as far as the superior aspect of the brachiocephalic vein.

Compartment 4[80]

Lymph nodes between the brachiocephalic vein and tracheal bifurcation within the anterior and posterior mediastinum.

Selective neck dissection

Any type of cervical lymphadenectomy which involves less than dissection of levels I–V where the spinal accessory nerve (SAN), the internal jugular vein (IJV) and sternocleidomastoid muscle (SCM) are preserved. The levels of node dissection should be clearly recorded.

Radical neck dissection

Radical neck dissections are very rarely indicated in the treatment of thyroid cancer but are defined here to ensure accuracy of nomenclature:

- A classical *radical neck dissection* removes all the lymphatic tissue in levels I–V along with the SAN, SCM and IJV.

- *Extended neck dissection* is defined as removal of one or more additional lymph node groups such as parapharyngeal, superior mediastinal and paratracheal nodes and/or non-lymphatic structures (digastric muscle, skin).

- *Modified radical neck dissection* (MRND) involves removal of lymph nodes in levels I–V with preservation of one or more non-lymphatic structures as follows:
  - *MRND Type I:* excision of all lymph nodes routinely removed by radical neck dissection with preservation of the SAN.
  - *MRND Type II:* excision of all lymph nodes routinely removed by radical neck dissection with preservation of the SAN and IJV.
  - *MRND Type III (functional or comprehensive neck dissection):* excision of all lymph nodes routinely removed by radical neck dissection with preservation of the SAN, IJV and SCM.

The type of surgery to be offered is straightforward in most cases and only requires endorsement by the MDT. In other complex cases the MDT must offer guidance on the basis of the individual patient's cytology and circumstances.

Surgery for papillary carcinoma

i   Patients with a node negative cancer of 1 cm diameter or less (pT1, section 1.4) can be adequately treated by lobectomy followed by levothyroxine therapy (section 8.3)[9,60,64,69,70,73] (III, B).

ii   For most patients, especially those with tumours greater than 1 cm in diameter, multifocal disease, extrathyroidal spread, familial disease and those with clinically involved nodes, total thyroidectomy is indicated[13,23] (III, B). Total thyroidectomy is also indicated where there is a history of previous neck irradiation in childhood (IV, C).

iii   If the diagnosis of thyroid cancer has been made after thyroid lobectomy and completion (contralateral) thyroid lobectomy is required; the latter should be offered within 8 weeks of histological diagnosis of cancer (IV, C).

iv   Lobectomy alone may be appropriate treatment for some patients with tumours larger than 1 cm in diameter if the MDT judges that the risk of recurrence is low (IV, C).

v   In patients with clinically uninvolved nodes but who are deemed high risk (ie they have any of the following features: male sex, age >45 years, tumours greater than 4 cm in diameter, extracapsular or extrathyroidal disease), total thyroidectomy *and* level VI node dissection should be performed[67,71] (IV, C).

vi   Palpable disease in level VI nodes discovered at surgery is treated by a level VI node dissection. When suspicious/clinically involved nodes are apparent pre-operatively or are encountered at surgery in the lateral neck, and confirmed by needle biopsy or frozen section, then a selective neck dissection (levels IIa–Vb) is recommended, preserving the accessory nerve, sternocleidomastoid muscle and internal jugular vein[28] (IV, C).

Surgery for follicular carcinoma

i   FNAC cannot at present distinguish follicular adenoma or benign hyperplastic nodules from carcinoma[62,66,81] (IV, C). Thy3 cytology usually mandates lobectomy as the least surgical procedure, although in some cases (identified by the descriptive report or by the specific clinical scenario) discussion at the MDT before deciding on an appropriate course of action may be indicated (section 3.1).

ii   Frozen section examination is unhelpful when the FNAC diagnosis is that of a follicular lesion (Thy3)[81] (IV, C).

iii   If definitive histology reveals a follicular adenoma or a hyperplastic nodule, no further treatment is required (III, B).

iv   A follicular carcinoma under 1 cm in diameter with minimal capsular invasion should be treated by lobectomy (section 8.3)[69,70,73] (IV, C).

v   Patients with follicular cancer showing evidence of vascular invasion should be treated with total thyroidectomy (IV, C).

vi   Patients with follicular carcinoma more than 4 cm in diameter should be treated with near-total or total thyroidectomy (C).

vii   Low-risk patients (females, patients <45 years of age) with tumours measuring <2 cm in diameter may be managed by lobectomy alone and levothyroxine therapy following MDT discussion and informed consent[70,82,83] (III, B).

viii   Clear recommendations for otherwise low-risk patients with tumours 2–4 cm in diameter showing minimal capsular invasion only cannot be made. Treatment should be at the discretion of the MDT (IV, C).

ix Palpable/suspicious cervical lymph nodes are dealt with in a similar manner to papillary carcinoma (see section above, points v and vi)[9,13,70] (IV, C).

x If the diagnosis of thyroid cancer has been made after thyroid lobectomy and completion, (contralateral) thyroid lobectomy is required; the latter should be offered within 8 weeks of histological diagnosis of cancer (IV, C).

Surgery for oncocytic follicular (Hürthle cell) carcinoma

Oncocytic follicular (Hürthle cell) carcinomas may behave more aggressively[71,84] than other histological types of DTC. Hürthle cell tumours are less likely to concentrate ^{131}I and total thyroidectomy should be considered.

Surgery for papillary or follicular microcarcinoma

Patients with DTCs less than 1 cm in diameter have an extremely low risk of death from thyroid cancer (0.1%)[18,85,86] and can therefore be treated adequately by thyroid lobectomy (III, B) provided that:

- the tumour does not extend beyond the thyroid capsule
- there is no evidence of metastases
- there is no evidence of vascular invasion
- there is no evidence of multifocality
- there is no evidence of contralateral disease.

5.3 Emergency surgery

It is rare for emergency surgery to be needed. Usually a careful work-up of patients is achievable. However, acute presentation of a patient with thyroid cancer and severe airway compromise requires urgent/immediate surgery (IV, C).

5.4 Surgery for locally advanced disease

i When pre-operative vocal cord examination has revealed no sign of recurrent laryngeal nerve involvement every attempt should be made to dissect the tumour from the nerve/s (IV, C). In patients with unilateral nerve involvement associated with extensive extrathyroidal disease, the nerve may have to be sacrificed to achieve a curative procedure.

ii It may not be possible to remove the entire tumour without damaging both recurrent laryngeal nerves. A small residue of tumour may be left behind to protect the nerve/s and be subsequently dealt with by ^{131}I ablation and suppression of thyroid-stimulating hormone (TSH) with levothyroxine (section 8.3), with or without external beam radiotherapy (section 7).[74]

iii In individual patients with locally advanced disease involving the upper aero-digestive tract and/or one or both recurrent laryngeal nerves, curative excisional surgery of the tracheal wall and/or oesophagus should be considered (IV, C).

iv When radical curative surgery is not possible or agreed to by the patient, treatment with radical radiotherapy and ^{131}I should be considered (IV, C).

5.5 Early post-surgical management

i   After total/near-total thyroidectomy, patients should be started on triiodothyronine (T3) (IV, C). Normal adult dosage is T3 20 mg tds. This should be stopped for two weeks before either a radioiodine scan or ^{131}I ablation of thyroid remnant (IV, C).

ii Serum calcium should be checked within 24 hours of surgery. If hypocalcaemia is detected, it should be treated as indicated in section 8.2 (III, B).

iii A baseline postoperative serum Tg should be checked, preferably no earlier than 6 weeks after surgery[55,87–91] (III, B).

5.6 Medullary thyroid cancer

The management of MTC is discussed in section 14.

5.7 Surgical management of other rare malignancies of the thyroid

Thyroid lymphoma

Primary thyroid lymphomas occur on a background of Hashimoto's thyroiditis in the vast majority of cases, although the Hashimoto's thyroiditis may be undiagnosed.

i   A clinical diagnosis or high index of suspicion of lymphoma may be confirmed by FNAC with the addition of molecular techniques, although usually a core biopsy is required to allow a full range of immunocytochemical studies to be performed.

ii Incision biopsy is not essential for the diagnosis of lymphoma[92] (III, B).

iii Thyroidectomy is not indicated[93] (III, B).

iv The treatment of choice is chemotherapy followed by radiotherapy or radiotherapy alone. Most cases are high-grade B cell lymphomas. Some are MALT (mucosa-associated lymphoid tissue) tumours.

v   Prognosis is generally excellent.

vi Patients should be referred to an MDT specialising in lymphoma management (IV, C).

Anaplastic thyroid cancer

This has a very poor prognosis.[94]

i   Where the diagnosis has not been possible on FNAC, core biopsy may assist the diagnosis.

ii Surgery is rarely indicated. In a very small subgroup of cases, chemotherapy/radiotherapy and surgery may achieve a slightly longer period of survival[94–96] (III, B).

iii ^{131}I ablation or therapy has no place (III, B).

iv External beam radiotherapy is the mainstay of treatment, with or without chemotherapy[94,96] (III, B).

6 Radioiodine ablation and therapy for differentiated thyroid cancer

Following a total or near-total thyroidectomy, some radioiodine uptake is usually demonstrable in the thyroid bed. ^{131}I-induced destruction of this residual thyroid tissue is known as 'radioiodine remnant ablation'. 'Radioiodine therapy' refers to administration of ^{131}I with the intention to treat recurrent or metastatic disease. The principles and procedures are similar for the administration of ^{131}I for ablation or therapy purposes; the latter is discussed further in section 9.1.

6.1 Preparation for ^{131}I ablation or therapy

i   The patient should be seen by an appropriate member of the MDT (an Administration of Radioactive Substances Advisory Committee (ARSAC) Certificate holder), preferably in a combined clinic, for assessment and full discussion about radioiodine studies and treatment. Informed consent must be obtained from the patient before treatment (**IV, C**).

ii Patients should adopt a low iodine diet for 2 weeks prior to ^{131}I and other sources of excess iodine should be eliminated (eg recent CT scan with contrast material) (see Appendix 5, patient information leaflet 3)[97–100](**III, B**). Amiodarone may have to be withdrawn for several months to ensure optimal conditions for ^{131}I ablation or therapy.

iii ^{131}I ablation and therapy must be given only in centres suitably equipped and certified for the purpose[101a] (**IV, C**).

iv If ^{131}I can be administered within 3–4 weeks of thyroidectomy, no thyroid hormone replacement is required in the interim period. This would usually allow TSH to rise to >30 mIU/L at the time of ablation. For most centres, however, the interval between thyroidectomy and ^{131}I ablation will be longer. In these circumstances, patients should start T3 20 mg tds following surgery; this should be stopped 2 weeks before planned ablation to allow the serum TSH to rise to >30 mIU/L (**IV, C**).

v   A pre-ablation scan is not indicated routinely. If there is doubt about completeness of surgery, a pre-ablation scan can be performed to assess remnant size. In such cases ^{123}I or ^{99m}Tc-pertechnetate may be preferable to ^{131}I in order to reduce the risk of stunning.[101,102] Demonstration of large thyroid remnants should lead to consideration of further surgery before ^{131}I ablation[103] (**III, B**).

vi **Pregnancy must be excluded before** [131]I **ablation or therapy** (**IV, C**).

vii Breastfeeding must be discontinued at least 4 weeks and preferably 8 weeks before ^{131}I ablation or therapy (**IV, C**) and should not be resumed.

viii Pre-treatment sperm banking should be considered in male patients likely to have more than two high-dose ^{131}I therapies[104,105] (**IV, C**). Adequate hydration at the time of treatment and for several days afterwards, regular emptying of the bladder and avoidance of constipation helps to prevent a decrease in sperm count.

6.2 Postoperative ^{131}I ablation

i   The 2002 edition of these guidelines recommended that most patients with DTC tumours greater than 1–1.5 cm in diameter should receive ^{131}I ablation. This was based on several retrospective studies,[13,32,36,106–108] including a large cohort study with long follow-up,[13] which showed that patients older than 45 years with tumours greater than 1.5 cm in diameter had reduced local and distant recurrence and cancer death rates after remnant ^{131}I ablation. This recommendation (III, B) remains largely valid; however, recent evidence suggests that the benefit of ^{131}I ablation for low-risk (section 1.4) patients may be questionable.[109,110]

ii   Furthermore, recent data indicate that the incidence of a second malignancy after radioiodine might be higher than previously thought.[111,112] In the light of these findings, the MDT decision about ^{131}I ablation should be individualised and selective (IV, C).

iii Factors other than size of tumour (such as presence of metastases, completeness of excision, age, degree of invasion, associated comorbidities) should be taken into account (IV, C).

iv   Patients should be counselled so that they understand the rationale for ^{131}I ablation (IV, C).

v   The benefits of ^{131}I ablation include:

- eradication of all thyroid cells including potential destruction of residual postoperative microscopic disease and thus possible reduced risk of local and distant tumour recurrence
- reassurance to patients imparted by the knowledge that serum Tg is undetectable and iodine scan negative, implying that all thyroid tissue has been destroyed
- possible prolonged survival[13,32]
- increased sensitivity of monitoring by serum Tg measurements and possibly earlier detection of recurrent or metastatic disease.[9,113]

vi   The acute and late side effects of radioiodine (also see section 6.4) should be discussed with the patient (IV, C), particularly stressing:

- moderate risk of a dry mouth and sialadenitis
- very small risk of second malignancies.

vii Whenever possible the patient should make an informed decision based on the above risks and benefits (IV, C).

In the absence of randomised trials, recommendations on ^{131}I ablation have to be based on retrospective studies[1,13,32,36,107,108,114] and recent consensus statements.[70,83]

Box 1. Indications, probable indications and lack of indications for ^{131}I ablation.

A. *No indication for ^{131}I ablation (low risk of recurrence or cancer-specific mortality)* **(III, B)**

Patients should satisfy all the criteria below for ^{131}I ablation to be omitted:

- complete surgery
- favourable histology
- tumour unifocal, ≤1cm in diameter, N0, M0, or minimally invasive FTCs, without vascular invasion smaller than 2 cm in diameter[82,83]
- no extension beyond the thyroid capsule.

B. *Definite indications* **(III, B)**

Any of the following criteria constitute an indication for ^{131}I ablation:

- distant metastases
- incomplete tumour resection
- complete tumour resection but high risk of recurrence or mortality (tumour extension beyond the thyroid capsule, or more than 10 involved lymph nodes and more than three lymph nodes with extracapsular spread.[113]

C. *Probable indications* **(IV, C)**

The list of indications below applies to patients who do not fall under categories A and B above. Any one of the following categories is a 'probable' indication for ^{131}I ablation:

- less than total thyroidectomy (inferred from operation notes or pathology report, or when an ultrasound scan or isotope scan shows a significant postoperative thyroid remnant)
- status of lymph nodes not assessed at surgery (section 5.2)
- tumour size >1 cm and <4 cm in diameter
- tumours <1 cm in diameter with unfavourable histology (tall-cell, columnar-cell or diffuse sclerosing papillary cancers, widely invasive or poorly differentiated follicular cancers)
- multifocal tumours <1 cm.[113,114]

Activity of ^{131}I for ablation

i   The present recommendation for remnant ablation is 3.7 GBq pending the results of ongoing trials[115,116] **(III, B)**.

ii   For patients with known metastases, higher ^{131}I activities (5–7.4 MBq)[117] are often used.

Procedure for remnant ablation with [131]I

i   Patient information leaflets (Appendix 5) and support from the specialist nurse should be provided **(IV, C)**.

ii   Serum TSH and Tg should be measured immediately prior to ^{131}I administration **(IV, C)**.

iii A pregnancy test *must* be performed where indicated, immediately prior to ^{131}I administration; the result should be negative **(IV, C)**.

iv   The serum TSH should be >30 mIU/L at the time of ablation (see section 6.1iv) **(IV, C)**.

v   Recombinant human TSH (rhTSH) has recently been licensed for remnant ablation after total or near-total thyroidectomy, based on a randomised controlled trial in low-risk (section 1.4) patients.[118] In cases where thyroxine withdrawal is contraindicated or ineffective in raising the serum TSH, rhTSH may also be used for ablation. Discussion of such cases by the MDT is recommended (**IV, C**). The protocol consists of 0.9 mg rhTSH administered intramuscularly on 2 consecutive days followed by 3.7 GBq of ^{131}I ablation 24 hours after the second rhTSH injection.

Aftercare following ^{131}I ablation

i   After admission for ^{131}I ablation, ward procedures should be followed and the patient discharged only after medical physics assessment. Written advice about restricting the extent of contact between the patient and others should be handed to the patient before discharge (**IV, C**). At the time of discharge (usually 3 days after ^{131}I), thyroid hormone treatment (normally levothyroxine) should be commenced and a letter must go to the GP with the patient (**IV, C**).

ii   A post-ablation scan should be performed 3–10 days after the ^{131}I dose[119] (**III, B**).

iii Patients should be reviewed (preferably in a combined clinic) after 2–3 months for assessment, adjustment of TSH suppressive dose of levothyroxine, and to make arrangements for follow-up Tg measurement and scanning (**IV, C**).

6.3   Diagnostic scan ([131]I 74–150 MBq)[98,120]

Indications for ^{131}I diagnostic scan after ^{131}I ablation

Diagnostic scans are carried out to assess the effectiveness of ablation or therapy and requirement for further ^{131}I therapy.[121]

Recent data indicate that low-risk cases (section 1.4) may be assessed adequately by measuring serum Tg (in the absence of Tg assay interference) under conditions of TSH stimulation, without the need for a radioiodine scan which rarely provides additional helpful information in such cases.[121–124] In low-risk cases, therefore, the diagnostic scan may be omitted, although TSH-stimulated serum Tg should be assessed. If a diagnostic scan is omitted, ultrasonography of the neck is a valuable alternative in assessing local recurrence (section 8.5).

A diagnostic radioiodine scan (in conjunction with stimulated serum Tg measurement) should be performed in all other cases[121] (**III, B**).

Indications for repeat diagnostic scans after radioiodine ablation

i   Patients with high-risk disease and with Tg antibodies (TgAb) interfering with serum Tg measurements may need additional radioiodine, ultrasound or other cross-sectional (eg CT or MRI) scans (section 8.5).

ii   No further diagnostic radioiodine scans are required for other groups of patients, unless there are indications of disease progression, such as a rising serum Tg, clinical or radio-logical evidence of progression (section 8.5). In such cases, scans should be performed after thyroid hormone withdrawal rather than rhTSH unless there are clear contraindications to thyroid hormone withdrawal (further discussed in section 8.5) (**III, B**).

Precautions

i   *Pregnancy:* ARSAC recommends a minimum period of 6 months before conception for females, as the absorbed dose to the fetus should not exceed 1 mGy[125] (III, C). If pregnancy is deferred for at least 6 months after high-dose ^{131}I ablation or therapy to the mother, there is no risk to the fetus. Fertility is not impaired though there is a slightly increased risk of miscarriage if pregnancy occurs within 1 year of high-dose ^{131}I ablation[126–129] (III, B).

ii In males, a 4-month period of avoidance of fathering a child is recommended[125] (IV, C).

Timing of radioiodine diagnostic scans

Diagnostic radioiodine scans are usually scheduled not earlier than 6 months after ^{131}I ablation. In selected cases (patients with aggressive disease), this should be brought forward to four months[119] (IV, C).

Procedure

i   Before a diagnostic radioiodine scan, patients should switch from levothyroxine to T3 replacement (T3 20 µg td). Levothyroxine is routinely stopped four weeks, and T3 two weeks before the diagnostic scan (IV, C).

ii The serum TSH and Tg should be measured on the day of the diagnostic scan and before the tracer dose of radioiodine is administered. A serum TSH >30 mIU/L is required for optimal imaging (IV, C).

iii If abnormal uptake of the tracer is detectable, further ^{131}I therapy (usually 3.7–5.5 GBq) should be given (IV, C). A post-treatment scan should be performed 3–10 days later, as it is a significantly more sensitive procedure than a diagnostic radioiodine scan employing a small (74-150 MBq) activity of [131]I [119] (section 9) (III, B).

iv Patients should restart levothyroxine when the scan has been reported and discussed with the patient. The dose of levothyroxine is the same as prior to the diagnostic scan. Levothyroxine should not be restarted earlier than three days after the diagnostic radioiodine scan. Caution should be exercised when recommencing levothyroxine in patients with vascular disease (IV, C).

v   A low iodine diet should be advised for 2 weeks before diagnostic radioiodine scans (and ^{131}I ablation or therapy) (section 6.1ii and Appendix 5, patient information leaflet 3) (III, B).

vi Patients should have access to the clinic, the ward where iodine treatment was given, a specialist nurse or the clinician's secretary (IV, C).

6.4   Short-term and long-term side effects of ^{131}I ablation and therapy

The main side effect is transient hypothyroidism, unless rhTSH is used[118, 123,130] (section 6.2).

Possible early effects

∎   Abnormality of taste and sialadenitis can be minimised by good hydration.

∎   Nausea is possible and can be minimised by antiemetics.

- Neck discomfort and swelling within a few days of radioiodine can occur but are rare. They are more common when a large thyroid remnant is present. Simple analgesics should be tried initially. A short course of steroids may be necessary in severe cases.

- Radiation cystitis, radiation gastritis, bleeding into secondary deposits and oedema in cerebral secondary deposits are all extremely rare after administered activities of 3 GBq or less.[100,104,113]

Possible late effects

- Dry mouth and abnormal taste may occur.

- Sialadenitis and lachrymal gland dysfunction may occur.

- Lifetime incidence of leukaemia and second cancers is low, affecting around 0.5% of patients.[100,131–133] Only one of three cohort studies showed an increased but non-significant risk of leukaemia (relative risk about 2). The risk of leukaemia increases with a high cumulative dose (greater than 18.5 GBq) and with use of additional external beam radiotherapy. Patients who have a high cumulative dose of ^{131}I may also be more likely to develop second malignancies (eg the bladder and possibly colorectal, breast and salivary glands).[111,112,131] The total cumulative activity should therefore be kept as low as possible.[106,107,131–136]

- Radiation fibrosis can occur in patients who have had diffuse pulmonary metastatic disease and have received repeated doses of [131]I.[136–138]

- Increased risk of miscarriage may persist for up to 1 year after ^{131}I ablation/therapy.[126–129]

- Infertility may occur in men.[104,105]

7 External beam radiotherapy

Postoperative adjuvant external beam radiotherapy is infrequently indicated for DTC. It probably reduces local recurrence in patients at high risk due to residual disease where further surgery is not appropriate.[96,139,140] Radiotherapy should be planned carefully, preferably using three-dimensional conformal planning techniques, with appropriate precautions taken for prevention of radiation myelopathy[15,107,141–145] (III, B).

Intensity modulated radiotherapy (IMRT) may have advantages over conventionally planned radiotherapy when treating the thyroid bed and regional nodes. However, an important consideration in the adjuvant setting is that the use of IMRT with multiple fields can theoretically increase the risk of second malignancies in long-term survivors.[146]

7.1 Adjuvant external beam radiotherapy

The main indications for adjuvant radiotherapy are:

i   gross evidence of local tumour invasion at surgery, presumed to have significant macro- or microscopic residual disease, particularly if the residual tumour fails to concentrate sufficient amounts of radioiodine

ii   extensive pT4 disease in patients over 60 years of age with extensive extranodal spread after optimal surgery, even in the absence of evident residual disease.[96,108,141,144–146]

7.2 High-dose external beam radiotherapy as part of primary treatment

High-dose external beam radiotherapy is indicated for (IV, C):

i   unresectable tumours that do not concentrate radioactive iodine

ii   unresectable bulky tumours in addition to radioactive iodine treatment.

For palliative radiotherapy, see section 9.2.

8 Post-treatment follow-up

Routine follow-up includes clinical assessment of thyroid status and examination of the neck or other relevant systems. Abnormal masses in the neck or elsewhere should trigger further investigations, which may include FNAC (**IV, C**).

8.1 Voice dysfunction

This may result if there is external laryngeal nerve and/or recurrent nerve injury.

i   Voice dysfunction must be investigated if symptoms persist beyond 2 weeks after surgery (**IV, C**).

ii   The patient should be referred to a specialist practitioner capable of carrying out direct and/or indirect laryngoscopy (**IV, C**).

8.2 Management of hypocalcaemia

i   Serum calcium should be checked on the day after surgery, and daily until the hypocalcaemia improves[147,148] (**III, B**). A decline in serum calcium concentration in the first 24 hours after surgery is predictive of the need for calcium supplementation.[149]

ii   If hypocalcaemia develops, calcium supplementation should be started at an initial dose of 500 mg elemental calcium three times daily (**IV, C**). The dose is adjusted as indicated by the response. Occasionally intravenous calcium gluconate may be required. Mild asymptomatic hypocalcaemia usually does not require treatment, although monitoring is indicated.

iii   If hypocalcaemia does not improve or worsens, introduce alfacalcidol (or calcitriol) (**III, B**).

iv   Close monitoring of serum calcium is needed to prevent hypercalcaemia (**IV, C**).

v   Monitoring of serum calcium should be supervised in the specialist clinic, with the assistance of the GP if appropriate (**IV, C**).

vi   After total thyroidectomy, 30% of patients will need calcium supplementation with or without alfacalcidol. By 3 months, less than 10% of patients will still require calcium supplementation.[150]

vii   Hypoparathyroidsm is often transient and a predictor of this is an elevated (or upper normal range) serum parathyroid hormone (PTH) concentration at the time of the occurrence of hypocalcaemia.[150] Thus, the majority of patients on calcitriol/alfacalcidol l/calcium supplements can have this treatment withdrawn. Supplements should be slowly and gradually reduced and serum calcium monitored every few months until withdrawn and eucalcaemia restored. The combined effects of hypocalcaemia and hypothyroidism are poorly tolerated and calcitriol/alfacalcidol/calcium supplement withdrawal should take place during euthyroidism (**IV, C**).

viii If hypoparathyroidism is permanent, the lowest dose of supplements should be administered to maintain the serum calcium at the lower end of the normal range, while avoiding hypercalciuria. In stable cases annual measurement of serum calcium is recommended (IV, C).

8.3 Long-term suppression of serum thyrotrophin

i Levothyroxine should be used in preference to T3 for long-term suppression[151] (III, B).

ii The dose of levothyroxine should be sufficient to suppress the TSH to <0.1 mIU/L[151–155] (III, B).

iii The dose of levothyroxine should be adjusted by 25 µg (every 6 weeks) until the serum TSH is <0.1 mIU/L) (IV, C). To achieve this, most patients will require 175 or 200 µg daily.

iv In patients with low-risk (section 1.4) DTC, there is some evidence that it may be adequate to keep the serum TSH below the reference range in the absence of full TSH suppression (typically 0.1–0.5 mIU/L)[151–155] (III, B), but robust long-term data are not available.

v Suppressive levothyroxine therapy is best supervised by a member of the MDT, preferably by an endocrinologist (IV, C), although alternative arrangements may be appropriate in low-risk cases (see section 10v).

vi The GP should be advised of the reason for this suppression and of the target serum TSH concentration (IV, C).

8.4 Measurement of serum thyroglobulin in long-term follow-up (Appendix 1)

Tg is secreted by both normal and cancerous thyroid cells. In patients who have not had a total thyroidectomy and ^{131}I ablation, the interpretation of serum Tg measurements is limited by the inability to differentiate between tumour and thyroid remnant.[156,157] Detectable serum Tg is highly suggestive of thyroid remnant, residual or recurrent tumour.

The cut-off serum Tg concentration beyond which recurrent/persistent disease is implied depends on several variables including the assay employed by each laboratory. Individual laboratories should advise clinicians on the significance of detectable serum Tg at low concentrations (Appendix 1) (IV, C).

A serum Tg rising with time while on suppressive thyroxine therapy is highly suggestive of tumour recurrence or progression.

Endogenous TgAb and other unidentified factors may interfere with the measurement of serum Tg. Measurement of TgAb is valuable in interpreting the serum Tg result, although the absence of TgAb does not absolutely exclude the possibility of interference with the Tg assay. There is evidence that TgAb measurement may be of some value in monitoring patients with thyroid cancer.[157]

i To ensure continuity in monitoring, clinicians should use the same laboratory and Tg assay on a long-term basis. Laboratories should not change methods without prior consultation with clinical users of the service (IV, C).

ii TgAb should be measured by a quantitative method simultaneously with measurement of serum Tg. If TgAb are detectable, measurement should be repeated at regular (~6-monthly) intervals. If negative, they should be measured at follow-up when Tg is measured[55] (IV, C).

iii Samples should not be collected sooner than 6 weeks post-thyroidectomy or ^{131}I ablation/therapy[55,156-161] (III, C).

iv There is normally no need to measure serum Tg more frequently than 3-monthly during routine follow-up; for patients in remission, an annual check of serum Tg should be measured while on suppressive levothyroxine treatment (IV, C).

v Since Tg release is TSH-dependent, serum TSH concentration should be determined concurrently to aid interpretation. The requesting clinician should indicate on the form whether the patient is on thyroid hormone therapy and the TSH result should be available to the laboratory performing the Tg assay (IV, C).

vi There is no need for TSH stimulation if the basal serum Tg is already detectable.

vii Patients in whom the basal Tg remains persistently detectable (ie while on suppressive levothyroxine therapy) or rises with subsequent assessments require further evaluation[157] (III, B).

viii At routine follow-up most patients should have serum Tg measured while on TSH suppression (IV, C).

TSH-stimulated serum Tg measurement

The diagnostic sensitivity of serum Tg measurements is enhanced by an elevated serum TSH concentration[156,157] Tumour recurrence or progression can be diagnosed earlier by detecting a raised serum Tg after TSH stimulation than by measurement of Tg on suppressive thyroxine therapy. Tg should be measured when the serum TSH is more than 30 mIU/L (usually in conjunction with diagnostic radioiodine scans) (IV, C).

In low-risk (section 1.4) patients who have undetectable serum Tg while on suppressive thyroxine therapy, stimulated serum Tg measurement alone (ie without a concomitant whole-body scan (WBS)) represents adequate initial follow-up, provided there is no Tg assay interference.[70,122,124] A concomitant WBS in such cases rarely adds valuable information, although ultrasonography of the neck may be indicated (section 8.5). If serum Tg is undetectable under TSH stimulation, then in low-risk patients subsequent long-term follow-up by measurement of serum Tg under TSH suppression alone is sufficient[70,122,124] (III, B).

TSH stimulation can be achieved either by thyroid hormone withdrawal (aiming for a serum TSH >30 mIU/L; section 6.3), or by injections of rhTSH while the patient remains on suppressive thyroxine therapy. The latter is indicated in selected cases (see below).

i TSH-stimulated serum Tg measurements (with or without a radioiodine scan) should be performed 6–8 months after ^{131}I ablation or therapy (IV, C). A single undetectable TSH-stimulated serum Tg in the absence of assay interference is highly predictive of no future recurrence provided the Tg can be measured reliably (ie with no assay interference) in low-risk (section 1.4) patients who have undergone total or near-total thyroidectomy and ^{131}I ablation.[162] The role of neck ultrasonography in such cases is discussed in section 8.5.

ii   The TSH-stimulated serum Tg may remain detectable at low concentrations after ^{131}I ablation. This could be indicative of residual/recurrent cancer, but in the majority of cases signifies the presence of thyroid remnant. An expectant policy in low-risk (section 1.4) cases is recommended with repeat TSH-stimulated Tg assessments at 6–12 month intervals (**IV, C**). In many cases, repeat assessments will reveal a gradual decline in stimulated serum Tg to the point of no detection; routine follow-up should then be resumed.

iii Patients in whom the stimulated serum Tg remains persistently detectable or rises with subsequent assessments require further evaluation (section 9.1) (**III, B**).

Recommendations for the use of rhTSH-stimulated Tg in routine follow-up

TSH stimulation for measurement of serum Tg (or for WBS) can be achieved by thyroid hormone withdrawal or by administration of rhTSH.

i   The suitability of patients for rhTSH should be assessed by the MDT (**IV, C**).

ii   For the groups of patients with the following conditions, rhTSH is the only possible or safe option for diagnostic purposes[163] and for ablation or therapy:

- hypopituitarism
- functional metastases causing suppression of serum TSH
- severe ischaemic heart disease
- previous history of psychiatric disturbance precipitated by hypothyroidism
- advanced disease/frailty.

iii Patients should be informed about the advantages and disadvantages of this diagnostic method compared with conventional thyroid hormone withdrawal (**IV, C**).

iv   In patients known to have anti-Tg antibodies interfering with the Tg assay it is preferable to perform diagnostic radioiodine scans after thyroid hormone withdrawal, rather than with rhTSH. The Tg data may be impossible to interpret and WBSs after thyroid hormone withdrawal are more sensitive than after rhTSH administration[123] (**III, B**).

v   rhTSH is known to cause a transient but significant rise in serum thyroid hormone concentrations if functioning thyroid tissue is present. Therefore, caution should be exercised in patients with large thyroid remnants (**IV, C**).

vi   rhTSH (two 0.9 mg doses) should be administered by deep intramuscular injection on days 1 and 2 and serum Tg measured on day 5[123] (**Ib, A**). Due consideration must be given to the practicalities of collecting, handling and analysis of radioactive samples and advice must be obtained from the relevant radiation, transport and health and safety authorities (**IV, C**).

vii rhTSH should not be used if basal (unstimulated) serum Tg is elevated or the patient is expected to have ^{131}I therapy (**IV, C**).

viii rhTSH should be used with care if there is known or suspected tumour close to the central nervous system. Steroid cover is recommended in such cases (**IV, C**).

8.5 Role of imaging by ultrasonography and whole-body ^{131}I scanning in routine follow-up

After total thyroidectomy and postoperative ^{131}I ablation, diagnostic WBSs have relatively low sensitivity in detecting residual or recurrent disease compared with measurement of serum Tg.[122–124,164] Evidence supporting a specific adjunctive role for ultrasonography (in addition to routine measurement of serum Tg), or its utility compared with other modes of follow-up, is at present sparse.[67]

Ultrasonography is a sensitive method for detection of residual disease in the thyroid bed and metastatic disease in lymph nodes; its sensitivity is higher than neck palpation. This technique is used routinely during follow-up in some centres, especially outside the UK. Ultrasonography may uncommonly suggest the presence of disease in the absence of a rise in serum Tg and may indicate the site of disease in those with a raised serum Tg. Ultrasonography may have a particular role when serum Tg measurements are unreliable because of the presence of assay interference.

i   A single diagnostic WBS performed 6–8 months (but not sooner than 6 months) after ^{131}I ablation is generally indicated except in those with low-risk (section 1.4) disease (see iii below). If this is negative, further WBS is not usually required, depending on results of monitoring by measurement of serum Tg[121] (III, B).

ii   If rhTSH is used for WBS (see section 8.4 for indications) the recommended protocol is as follows[123] (Ib, A):

   ▪ rhTSH (0.9 mg) should be administered by deep intramuscular injection on days 1 and 2.

   ▪ A tracing dose of [131]I (approximately 150 MBq) should be given on day 3.

   ▪ The scan should be performed on day 5. A minimum of 30 minutes scanning time or a minimum of 140,000 counts per minute should be obtained.

   ▪ Serum Tg is also measured on day 5.

iii   Low-risk patients (section 1.4) who have been shown to have undetectable stimulated serum Tg in the absence of assay interference do not require routine diagnostic WBS during follow-up if the serum Tg on suppressive levothyroxine therapy remains undetectable. In such cases ultrasonography of the neck 6–12 months after thyroidectomy is indicated[122–124,164] (III, B).

iv   Patients who are likely to require ^{131}I therapy should have a WBS under conventional thyroid hormone withdrawal. This includes patients with detectable serum Tg, known thyroid remnant or known metastatic disease (IV, C).

9 Recurrent/persistent differentiated thyroid cancer

Early detection of recurrent disease can lead to cure or certainly long-term survival, particularly if the disease is operable or takes up radioactive iodine.[9,13,69,70,87,106,113,142,143,165] Distant metastases develop in 5–23% of patients with DTC, mainly in the lungs and bones.

Detection of abnormal masses in the neck or elsewhere should lead to FNAC and other appropriate investigations (IV, C).

9.1 Recurrence in the thyroid bed or cervical lymph nodes

Surgical re-exploration is the preferred method of management, usually followed by ^{131}I therapy[68,107] (III, B). Recurrent neck disease uncontrolled by surgery and ^{131}I therapy is best treated by high-dose palliative external beam radiotherapy (section 9.7). As patients are likely to survive for a significant period, radical external beam radiotherapy (doses 50–66 Gy) is often necessary with a daily fractionation and meticulous radiotherapy planning techniques.[96,139]

While the strategy outlined above is applicable in high-risk cases, the efficacy of an aggressive approach in low-risk cases where sensitive diagnostic techniques (high-definition ultrasonography, stimulated serum Tg measurements) indicate very low volume disease in the neck is less well established.

9.2 Metastatic disease involving lung and other soft tissue areas

These sites of metastases are usually not amenable to surgery and should be treated with ^{131}I therapy[13,100,136,166,167] (III, B). If the tumour takes up radioiodine, long-term survival is possible in such cases. The preferred treatment is repeated doses of ^{131}I; activities ranging from 3.7–10.1 GBq at 3–9 month intervals have been employed, the usual being 5.5 GBq given every 4–6 months until ^{131}I uptake is no longer evident.[98,136,142,166,167] Late side effects of ^{131}I therapy are minimised if intervals between treatments are no less than 6–12 months. While empirical doses are generally used, dosimetric assessment has also been helpful in certain studies.[96,167–169]

Pulmonary fibrosis following treatment with ^{131}I for diffuse pulmonary metastases has been reported rarely. It can be avoided or minimised by using an activity delivered less than 2.96 GBq (80 mCi) 48 hours after administration.[168]

There is no maximum limit to the cumulative ^{131}I dose that can be given to patients with persistent disease.[136] A normal blood count must be confirmed prior to each ^{131}I therapy administration and impairment of renal function would demand a lower dose[142] (IV, C).

A WBS 3–10 days after ^{131}I administration provides better scintigraphic assessment of disease than a diagnostic scan and response to treatment, although this has been questioned.[119]

9.3 Bone metastases

Extensive bony metastases are generally not curable by ^{131}I therapy alone. For solitary or limited number of bony metastases that are not cured by ^{131}I therapy, external beam radiotherapy with/without resection and/or embolisation should be considered in selected cases (IV, C). External beam radiotherapy also has a very important role in the management of spinal cord compression for vertebral metastases in addition to surgery.[96]

9.4 Cerebral metastases

External beam radiotherapy has an important palliative role in the management of cerebral metastases along with surgery if appropriate.[96]

9.5 Other metastatic sites

In selected cases when there are a limited number of metastases, metastasectomy or radiofrequency ablation may be helpful.

9.6 Unknown metastatic sites

For patients with rising serum Tg (section 8.4) and a negative diagnostic radioiodine scan the following checks are recommended[170] (III, B):

i   Ensure that the diagnostic ^{131}I scan is truly negative rather than falsely positive Tg (eg suboptimal serum TSH elevation).

ii Ensure that the Tg measurement is reliable and that there is no interference, particularly by heterophil antibodies.[171]

iii Check for possible iodine contamination (eg amiodarone therapy, or recent CT scan with contrast material).

The management of patients with a rising serum Tg and negative diagnostic radioiodine scan needs to be tailored to the individual after discussion in the MDT. There are three potential approaches:

(a) no action until the patient becomes symptomatic

(b) additional investigations aiming to localise the disease recurrence and offer specific therapy

(c) empirical use of ^{131}I therapy.[9,170,172,173]

If option (b) is judged to be appropriate, the following investigations are recommended:

i   Neck ultrasound (with or without FNAC), or cervico-mediastinal MRI scan should be performed as the most common sites of recurrence are the thyroid bed and cervical and mediastinal lymph nodes[124,164] (III, B).

ii If (i) is negative, a CT scan of the lungs without contrast should be done to exclude micronodular lung metastases (IV, C).

iii If (ii) is negative, then bony secondary deposits should be excluded, either by ^{99m}Tc bisphosphonate scan or, if indicated, other imaging agents like ^{99m}Tc MIBI (IV, C).

iv If the above are all negative, consider scanning with [18]fluoro-deoxy-glucose (FDG)-positron emission tomography (PET), [201]Thallium or ^{99m}Tc tetrofosmin, to exclude potentially operable disease. [18]FDG-PET scanning has a higher sensitivity for detecting dedifferentiating recurrent disease but at present is only available in selected centres in the UK.[174–178] Thyroxine withdrawal[175] and rhTSH administration[179] have been shown to increase the sensitivity of [18]FDG-PET scan. Patients with positive [18]FDG-PET scan have been shown to have a markedly reduced three-year survival compared with [18]FDG-PET scan-negative patients.[174] [18]FDG-PET scan may reveal recurrent disease which is operable. If the recurrent disease is not operable, consideration should be given to high-dose palliative external beam radiotherapy.

v ^{111}In octreotide imaging may be positive in some Tg positive iodine scan negative patients.[180] Data for the use of therapy with radiolabelled somatostatin analogues in patients with oncocytic follicular (Hürthle cell) carcinoma and dedifferentiated papillary carcinoma are limited.[181]

vi If all the above are still negative, therapeutic ^{131}I may be considered if the Tg continues to rise. Other factors that should be considered in making this decision include the risk category of the patient and the rate of rise of the serum Tg concentration.[182] In such cases a post-treatment scan (3–10 days after ^{131}I therapy) should be included as previously undetected metastases may then be visible. A recent meta-analysis of published studies confirms that 50% of post-therapy scans performed with 'blind' therapy will be positive and a fall in Tg levels will subsequently be observed in 60% of patients with positive post-therapy scans.[172] The usual dose of ^{131}I is 3–5.5 GBq. The decision to treat should be taken by the MDT with the full informed consent of the patient and consideration of the potential risks and benefits of the treatment in the absence of prospective randomised studies[83,183] (IV, C).

vii The combination of a positive diagnostic radioiodine scan and an undetectable serum Tg is very rare. In such cases the possibility of false positivity should be adequately explored before administering further ^{131}I therapy[184] (III, B).

9.7 Palliative care

Palliative care is not necessary in the vast majority of patients with DTC because they are cured. However, in a very small proportion of patients with recurrent end-stage disease (and in patients with anaplastic thyroid cancer) specialist palliative care would be necessary. A consultant in palliative medicine should liaise with the MDT and patients requiring palliative care referred early to the local palliative care team[185] (IV, C).

High-dose palliative external beam radiotherapy may be appropriate in good performance status patients with anticipated survival of more than 6 months. External beam radiotherapy also has a role in palliation of symptoms from fungating lymph nodes, bleeding tumour, stridor, superior vena caval obstruction and dysphagia.

Stridor and fear of choking are very distressing and can also be alleviated by pharmacological means, palliative surgery and counselling.

Palliative chemotherapy

Palliative chemotherapy may have a role in end-stage disease uncontrolled by surgery, ^{131}I therapy or external beam radiotherapy. The agents used are doxorubicin and cisplatinum, but durable responses are uncommon.[186,187] Chemotherapy should be used only in patients with progressive and symptomatic disease (**IV, C**). Concurrent chemo/radiotherapy has been tried, particularly in anaplastic carcinoma, with some very short-term benefits.[68,134,188,189] New treatments are coming online based upon an emerging understanding of the pathobiology of the disease. Agents that target different pathways are being developed and evaluated in clinical trials, and it may be appropriate to offer a patient with advanced disease the opportunity of participating in such a trial.

10 Long-term follow-up of differentiated thyroid cancer

i   Regular follow-up of DTC is necessary particularly for detection of early recurrence, initiation of appropriate treatment, TSH suppression and management of hypocalcaemia. This can be undertaken by a member of the MDT, working in a multidisciplinary setting and according to the established local guidelines (**IV, C**).

ii Once the thyroid remnant has been ablated, the frequency of attendance will be decided in each case individually: usually 3–6 monthly for the first 2 years, decreasing to 6–8 monthly for 3 years, and annually thereafter (**IV, C**).

iii Support and counselling may be necessary, particularly for younger patients, and in relation to pregnancy.

iv Follow-up should be lifelong (**IV, C**) for the following reasons:

  ■ The disease has a long natural history.

  ■ Late recurrences can occur, which can be successfully treated with a view to cure or long-term survival.

  ■ The consequences of supraphysiological levothyroxine replacement (such as atrial fibrillation and osteoporosis) need monitoring, especially as the patient ages.

  ■ Late side effects of ^{131}I treatment may develop, such as leukaemia or second tumours.

v   Low-risk cases who have completed their treatment, are shown to be free of disease at five years and no longer judged to require TSH suppression, may be followed up in settings other than the multidisciplinary thyroid cancer clinic. This may include a nurse-led clinic or primary care following agreement of well defined protocols and re-referral pathways.

vi At each visit the following tasks should be completed (**IV, C**):

  ■ Patient history should be taken.

  ■ A clinical examination should be performed.

  ■ Adequacy of TSH suppression and possible effects of thyrotoxicosis should be assessed.

  ■ Tg should be measured as a marker of tumour recurrence. *TgAb should be measured simultaneously with measurement of Tg.*[55]

  ■ The calcium status should be assessed in patients receiving treatment for hypoparathyroidism (**IV, C**).

11 Pregnancy and thyroid cancer

11.1 Diagnosis of thyroid cancer in pregnancy

The management of thyroid cancer diagnosed during pregnancy requires careful consideration of risks to mother and fetus. Thyroid cancer discovered during pregnancy does not behave more aggressively than that diagnosed in a similar aged group of non-pregnant women. Women of childbearing age with thyroid cancer generally have a good prognosis, similar to that of non-pregnant women.[190] Discussion of the case by the MDT, as well as counselling of the couple, are imperative (**IV, C**).

Surgery is indicated, but evidence regarding the optimum timing is unclear. Thyroidectomy in the first trimester of pregnancy carries a high risk of abortion, but may be performed safely in the second trimester. Alternatively, surgery can be deferred until after delivery, provided that the tumour is monitored regularly (eg by ultrasound) and found to be reasonably stable. In cases of advanced or aggressive disease delays in treatment would be undesirable, and termination of pregnancy may (rarely) need to be considered.

[131]I ablation or therapy must be avoided in pregnancy. Suppressive thyroxine therapy is safe during pregnancy.

   i   A thyroid nodule presenting during pregnancy should be investigated by FNAC (**IV, C**).

   ii   Radioiodine scans are contraindicated in pregnancy and during breastfeeding (**IV, C**).

   iii   If thyroid cancer is diagnosed or suspected, the following options should be considered (**IV, C**):

- Defer thyroidectomy, ^{131}I studies and treatment until the postpartum period.

- Perform a thyroidectomy during the second trimester of pregnancy, to be followed by suppressive doses of levothyroxine, but defer ^{131}I studies until the postpartum period.

- Termination of pregnancy followed by thyroidectomy and ^{131}I studies and treatment (this option is very rarely necessary).

11.2 Pregnancy in the treated patient

   i   In accordance with ARSAC, it is recommended that women should defer attempting conception for a minimum of 6 months and men for a period of 4 months following ^{131}I ablation or therapy[125] (**IV, C**). A small risk of spontaneous abortion may persist for up to 1 year after high-dose ^{131}I ablation or therapy.[126–128,131,190,191] There is no risk of previous ^{131}I ablation or therapy to the fetus, provided the recommendations are followed.[128,191]

   ii   Suppressive levothyroxine therapy should continue during pregnancy and to achieve this, the dose should be increased by approximately 25% as soon as pregnancy is confirmed[192] and further adjusted if necessary according to monitoring of TFTs (**III, B**).

iii The thyroid status should be checked by measurements of serum TSH and free thyroxine during each trimester to ensure that TSH remains suppressed, as levothyroxine requirements may increase during pregnancy[55,192] (IIa, B).

iv For men there should be a minimum period of 4 months from ^{131}I ablation or therapy before unprotected intercourse takes place[125] (IV, C).

12 Thyroid cancer in childhood

DTC is rare in children. Children at particular risk are those previously exposed to radiotherapy to the head or neck. Thyroid nodules are more likely to be malignant in children than in adults so surgical excision may be appropriate even if findings from FNAC suggest benign disease. Thyroid cancer in children aged 10 years or less is more aggressive than in adults and risk of recurrence is higher.[193,197]

i   The general principles of management are similar to those in adults; however, the managing team must include a paediatric endocrinologist, paediatric oncologist (or nuclear medicine physician) and nurse specialist or counsellor (**IV, C**).

ii Total thyroidectomy followed by TSH suppression is recommended for most patients[2] (**IV, C**).

iii Selective neck dissection is recommended for children with clinically positive neck nodes.[195]

iv ^{131}I ablation[2,195–197] is recommended for all children particularly those aged under 10 years, but the decision about ^{131}I ablation should be individually determined (**IV, C**).

v   Follow-up with serial serum Tg measurements should be lifelong[198] (**III, B**).

Guidelines for the management of DTC and MTC in children are available.[2]

MTC in children is also discussed in section 14.

13 Pathology reporting, grading and staging of thyroid cancers

13.1 General principles

Pathologists dealing with thyroid tumours should have a special interest in thyroid pathology or participate in a network with the opportunity of pathology review (IV, C). Many of the features affect staging and prognosis and may therefore influence clinical management decisions. A general approach to specimen handling is outlined below. Points specifically relating to medullary carcinoma are discussed in Section 14.

 i Cases should be handled and reported according to the datasets of the Royal College of Pathologists (RCPath)[199] (IV, C).

 ii Most lesions should have had FNAC before surgery (section 3)[49,69] (III, B), so at least a differential diagnosis should be available.

 iii Frozen section may be used to confirm the diagnosis of papillary carcinoma, but should not be used to differentiate follicular carcinoma from adenoma[199a,200] (Ib, A).

 iv In all cases, the blocks taken should be appropriate to make the diagnosis, and to assess the extent of invasion and the completeness of excision (IV, C).

 v Follicular lesions not grossly invasive should be widely sampled at the interface between the tumour, the capsule and the normal gland to detect capsular or vascular invasion. Small lesions (≤30 mm in maximum dimension) should be processed in their entirety and 10 blocks should be taken from larger lesions[30,201] (III, B, IV, C).

 vi Lymph nodes should be carefully dissected, the numbers counted and locations noted if possible (IV, C). Ipsilateral, midline and contralateral nodes should be documented separately (IV, C). Formal neck dissections should be dealt with according to RCPath protocols for head and neck cancers[203] (IV, C).

13.2 Gross description

A gross description should include the following features (IV, C):

▪ **Nature of specimen**	lobectomy	right or left
		total/near-total or subtotal
		± isthmus
	thyroidectomy	total or near-total
▪ **Weight and dimensions**		
▪ **Description of lesion(s)**	single or multifocal	
	solid or cystic	
	dimensions (of largest if multifocal)	
	encapsulated or not	
	confined to gland or invading adjacent structures	
▪ **Lymph nodes**	site	
	number	
	macroscopic involvement	

▪ **Presence or absence of parathyroid glands**

13.3 Microscopic report

The microscopic report should include the information listed below (IV, C).

Core datasets for all tumour types

▮ Type of carcinoma

▮ Whether the tumour is a single lesion or multifocal

▮ Maximum dimension of carcinoma

▮ Completeness of excision

▮ Extension into extrathyroidal tissues (which defines the lesion as pT4)

▮ Presence and extent of any lymphatic/vascular invasion

▮ Site and number of lymph nodes involved.

Additional points for histological subtypes

Papillary	Typical or variant (specify)	
Follicular	Angioinvasive or capsule only	Minimally invasive or widely invasive
Oncocytic (Hürthle cell) follicular carcinoma	(At least 75% Hürthle cells)	Report in same manner as follicular

13.4 Pathological staging

i   There are a number of classifications in current use for the staging of thyroid cancer.[202] It is recommended that at present pathological staging should be performed on the basis of TNM classification[202,204,205] (III, B). This is easy to apply and has been shown in a number of studies to correlate with outcome[10,196] (section 1.4).

ii The recommended stratification for age at diagnosis as under 45 years or 45 years and over should be applied to papillary and follicular tumours (IV, C).

iii In multifocal lesions, the largest is used for staging purposes (IV, C).

13.5 Staging protocol

See section 1.4.

13.6 Grading of tumours

i   Papillary carcinomas should have their specific subtype documented (eg classical, tall cell variant, etc) (IV, C).

ii Histological grading of thyroid tumours is not commonly performed and is not included in the RCPath dataset. However, grading may provide useful additional prognostic information.[27,206] It is therefore recommended that, where possible, a grade be assigned to the primary tumour as follows (IV, C):

G1   Well differentiated
G2   Moderately well differentiated
G3   Poorly differentiated
G4   Undifferentiated
GX   Grade cannot be assessed

39

For papillary tumours, a simple grading system based on a combination of marked nuclear atypia, tumour necrosis and vascular invasion has recently been proposed.[206] Grade 1 tumours have none of these features; Grade 2 have one or more. For follicular tumours, the presence of an insular, solid or other less well-differentiated component in a predominantly follicular lesion would warrant Grade 2. Predominance of the dedifferentiated component would place the tumour in Grade 3.

14 Management of medullary thyroid cancer

MTC is a rare disease (accounting for 5–10% of all thyroid cancers) that requires a dedicated, multidisciplinary regional service. All patients with MTC should be referred for surgical treatment to a cancer centre[5] (IV, C).

Developments in the molecular genetics of MTC have facilitated a rational framework for management. The use and interpretation of molecular diagnostics are difficult and require careful application in individual patients and their families.[207,208]

The biology of MTC has unique implications for the development and structure of clinical services and management of this unusual disease.

i   Twenty-five per cent of MTC is familial (multiple endocrine neoplasia 2A (MEN2A), MEN2B and familial medullary thyroid cancer (FMTC)), necessitating a comprehensive and integrated approach to both the patient and their family. The familial forms are inherited in an autosomal dominant manner.

ii   When MTC arises as part of a familial syndrome, assessment and management of the other endocrine tumours are required.

iii Patients may survive for many years even with a significant tumour burden. This makes the risk/benefit decisions for additional intervention for persistent or recurrent disease difficult.

iv   Clinical services for MTC should dovetail with those for MEN1 and MEN2, which require similar services and raise common issues (IV, C).

14.1 History

i   MTC may present with a lump in the neck or metastasis, or dysphagia, or with the systemic effects that result from coincident secretion of calcitonin and other peptides (frequent loose stools and vasomotor flushing). Less commonly, adrenocorticotrophin is secreted.

ii   The diagnosis may be made following FNAC of a thyroid nodule or lymph node in the absence of previous clinical suspicion. Unsuspected MTC can also be found at surgery.

iii In all cases, a comprehensive family history must be taken to include first- and second-degree relatives to search for features of MTC or other endocrinopathies that may occur in individuals with MEN2. This includes a history of unexpected sudden death, which should raise the suspicion of occult phaeochromocytoma[209,210] (IV, C).

14.2 Hospital investigation

Pre-operative investigations should include:

i   A baseline value for calcitonin[55,211,212] (Appendix 1, section 2) (III, B).

ii At least one 24-hour urine sample assayed for catecholamines and metanephrines to exclude phaeochromocytoma, and a serum calcium to exclude hyperparathyroidism.[212,213] These tests should be performed in all MTC patients prior to neck surgery even in the absence of a positive family history or symptoms (III, B).

iii *RET* mutation analysis to establish the possible genetic basis for the disease within an individual or kindred (III, B).

iv A stimulation test with calcium/pentagastrin may be indicated to confirm a diagnosis of MTC pre-operatively in relatives of patients with familial MTC, to exclude the rare causes of false-positive basal calcitonin elevation, or when calcitonin levels are only mildly elevated (Appendix 1).[55,156]

Routine pre-operative staging of MTC with ultrasound CT/MRI (chest, thorax, abdomen) is not essential *prior* to first-time intervention as it does not alter the need for neck surgery. These investigations, however, may provide the surgeon with information to guide the extent of surgery in the central compartment of the neck and superior mediastinum.

14.3 Treatment

Prior to thyroid surgery all patients should be managed as described in Section 5.1.

Surgery[207-209,214-217]

The aims of first-time surgical treatment of MTC are loco-regional control (the neck and superior mediastinum), and in some patients to obtain a biochemical as well as clinical cure.

i All patients with established MTC should undergo total thyroidectomy and central compartment node dissection. the inferior limit of the dissection being the brachiocephalic vein (levels VI and VII)[218] (III, B).

ii Patients with pT2–4 tumours, or palpable lymph nodes in the central or lateral compartment should in addition undergo bilateral selective neck dissection of levels IIa–Vb[218] (III, B).

iii In the absence of direct invasion, the sternomastoid muscle/internal jugular vein/accessory nerve should be conserved. Routine dissection of levels I, IIb and Va is not required unless there are palpable/suspicious nodes at these sites. The management of recurrent laryngeal nerve involvement by tumour is described in section 5. When there is strong suspicion or evidence of mediastinal node involvement below the brachiocephalic vein, the patient should be considered for further surgery (IV, C). This will require a sternotomy.[218]

iv Patients with distant metastases at presentation often have prolonged survival. Even in the presence of disseminated disease, surgery (total thyroidectomy and central compartment node dissection) should be considered to prevent subsequent compromise of the trachea, oesophagus and recurrent laryngeal nerves. These structures should be preserved whenever possible (IV, C).

v Prophylactic surgery should be offered to *disease-free* carriers of germ line *RET* mutations, identified by genetic screening programmes[216,219–221] (III, B). The possibility of future surgery should be discussed with parents before testing children (IV, C).

vi   In ideal circumstances these patients would be expected to have C-cell hyperplasia (CCH) rather than MTC but, in many cases, by the time of presentation the transition from CCH to MTC will have occurred. It is important to distinguish the need for therapeutic surgery from prophylactic surgery. This will depend upon the genotype, the age of the patient and the basal calcitonin.[219,222,223]

vii Children with MEN2B should undergo prophylactic thyroidectomy within the first year of life. Children with MEN2A should undergo prophylactic thyroidectomy before the age of 5 years[207,221] (III, B).

viii In children with MEN2A under the age of 10, it may be unnecessary to perform lymph node dissection. In older children and those with MEN2B, central compartment lymphadenectomy should probably be performed at the time of thyroidectomy.

ix   Gene carriers from kindred with FMTC should undergo prophylactic thyroid surgery after the age of 10; lymph node dissection is not indicated before the age of 20 years[222] (III, B).

x   Following surgery, voice dysfunction and hypocalcaemia should be managed as described in sections 8.1 and 8.2.

Investigation of persistent or increasing hypercalcitoninaemia

Postoperative samples should be measured no earlier than 10 days after thyroidectomy[55,224] (III, B). Plasma calcitonin levels are most informative 6 months after surgery.[55]

There is good evidence that meticulous initial surgery will reduce the risk of postoperative calcitonin elevation, but high calcitonin levels after surgery are a common finding. This will depend upon the pre-operative basal calcitonin, the stage of the tumour at presentation and the adequacy of initial surgery.[225,226]

True local recurrence is unusual after adequate initial surgery. When initial surgery was incomplete, re-operation on the neck (lymphadenectomy of the central and/or lateral compartments) with curative intent should be considered (IV, C).

Mediastinal lymphadenectomy may be necessary when there is a strong suspicion of, or proven nodal disease at this site.

It is important to distinguish loco-regional, persistent/recurrent disease from distant micro- or macro-metastases as the cause of an elevated calcitonin. Non-invasive imaging (chest and abdominal CT or MRI and cervical and/or abdominal ultrasound, bone scan) should be performed (IV, C) but may not be helpful because of the morphological pattern of metastatic MTC in lung and liver (ie miliary disease). Laparoscopy[227] or selective arteriography[228] will in some cases identify occult hepatic metastases. Other less invasive options to detect metastatic MTC in patients with rising calcitonin and negative whole-body CT or MRI include pentavalent ^{99m}Tc-dimercaptosuccinic acid (DMSA), ^{131}I-MIBG, ^{111}In-octreotide and ^{18}FDG-PET scans.

Re-operative surgery in the neck and mediastinum should be considered, even when there are known distant metastases, to prevent the complications of large volume disease affecting the airway, oesophagus or laryngeal nerves (IV, C).

Radiotherapy and chemotherapy

i   Routine adjuvant external beam radiotherapy has not been shown to improve survival[229,230] but may improve the relapse-free rate if there is gross microscopic residual disease or extensive nodal disease.[166,230]

ii   Radiotherapy may control local symptoms in cases of inoperable or secondary disease.

iii   Chemotherapy is generally ineffective, but may be tried for progressive and symptomatic disseminated disease.[96,186,187,230,231]

iv   Radiolabelled somatostatin analogue and/or ^{131}I-MIBG therapy may be useful in a small number of cases,[233–235] but have not been evaluated in clinical trials. Alpha-interferon and other new drugs may also have a role; however, the evidence base is scanty at present.

v   The use of suicide gene therapy and tyrosine kinase inhibitors is under investigation.[236,237]

vi   Treatment with any of these modalities should preferably take place within a clinical trial.

Palliative care

i   Medical therapy should concentrate on symptom control (IV, C).

ii   Gastrointestinal symptoms often respond well to symptomatic treatment (such as co-phenotrope and/or codeine phosphate). Somatostatin analogues are a possible alternative which may decrease tumour peptide release.

14.4 Follow-up

Lifelong follow-up is recommended (IV, C):

i   Response to primary surgery can be assessed clinically and by the measurement of serum calcitonin and tumour markers, usually 6 months after surgery[55] (IV, C).

ii   The presence of an elevated but stable calcitonin level postoperatively may be managed conservatively, provided treatable disease has been excluded radiologically. Progressively rising levels should trigger imaging for further staging. In the absence of recurrent symptoms, appropriate follow-up intervals are 6–12 months (IV, C).

14.5 Pathology

The general principles for specimen handling and gross description outlined in sections 13.1 and 13.2 should apply also to cases of medullary carcinoma. However, in cases of intrathyroidal tumour, the whole specimen should be blocked. Where possible, the upper third of the lobe(s) should be sampled and immunostained for calcitonin to identify CCH (IV, C).

Microscopic report

The general principles of section 13.3 apply. It is recommended that the diagnosis is confirmed by calcitonin immunoreactivity (IV, C).

The following features should also be noted (IV, C):

- presence of amyloid
- CCH.

Tumour staging

The staging protocols used in section 1.4 should be applied (**IV, C**). Age is not a prognostic factor in MTC.

Table 2. Medullary carcinoma staging.

Stage I	pT1, N0, M0
Stage II	pT2, N0, M0
	pT3, N0, M0
	pT4, N0, M0
Stage III	Any pT, N1, M0
Stage IV	Any pT, any N, M1

14.6 Molecular genetics[209,221,238–247]

Summary

i   It is important to recognise the heritable forms of MTC because of the risk of other tumours in the individual and the family. Early recognition and prophylactic surgery in MEN2 are effective in reducing both mortality and morbidity.

ii Approximately 25% of MTCs are hereditary, as part of the MEN2/FMTC syndrome.

iii Lack of family history does not exclude heritable disease. The disease may not be apparent in relatives because of 'skipped' generations, or an isolated case may be the start of a new family.

iv Inherited MTC without other endocrinopathies also occurs. It is inherited in similar ways but tends to be more indolent than other forms of MTC.[248]

v   Because of the rarity of MTC and the complexity of genetic investigation and management, cases should be managed by a specialist clinical service in close liaison with a regional genetics centre (**IV, C**).

Genetic investigation of a patient with MTC

1 Clinical history

A clinical history that is suggestive of MEN2 syndrome would include:

- symptoms/history of phaeochromocytoma, parathyroid disease
- features of MEN2B: facies (see Appendix 2), constipation/diarrhoea, presence of mucosal neuromas, medullated corneal nerve fibres, marfanoid habitus, colonic ganglioneuromatosis
- Hirschsprung's disease (occasionally associated with MEN2).

A systematic family history should be taken, to include all first- and second-degree relatives, with attention to features suggestive of MEN2 (thyroid, adrenal, parathyroid disease) (**IV, C**).

The history must be recorded in the case notes (**IV, C**).

2 Genetic testing

Before testing

i   If expertise is not available within the primary clinical team, the patient should be referred to the clinical genetics service (**IV, C**).

ii Because of the possibility of heritable disease, every case of MTC should be offered genetic testing unless there are good reasons for not undertaking this (**IV, C**).

iii Testing should always begin with the affected individual, if they are available (**IV, C**).

iv If the affected individual is not available, the decision and strategy for testing should be discussed with the clinical genetics service (**IV, C**).

v   Before blood is taken, a clear explanation must be given of the nature of the test, the possible outcomes, and of the implications of a positive or negative result for the individual and the family. This explanation should be recorded in the case notes for each individual (**IV, C**).

Testing

i   Ideally 10 ml EDTA anticoagulated blood should be taken from the affected individual. Tests can be performed on smaller (eg 1–2 ml) amounts of blood, but this should be discussed with the appropriate NHS genetics laboratory.

ii The sample together with clinical details and family history should be sent to the appropriate NHS genetics laboratory.

iii Patients with no special clinical features should be tested first for *RET* mutations in exons 10 and 11; if these are negative, for exons 13–16[243–247] (**III, B**). Failure to screen exons 13–16 constitutes an incomplete test.

iv Patients with clinical features of MEN2B should be tested first for mutations in codons 918 and 922 (exon 16), 883 (exon 15) and 804 and 806 (exon 14) (**IV, C**).

v   Patients with clinical features of Hirschsprung's disease should be tested first for mutations in codons 609, 611, 618, 620 (exon 10) (**IV, C**).

Action on results

If a mutation is found

i   The result should be communicated, in the clinic, to the patient (**IV, C**).

ii Permission must be obtained from the patient to disclose this result to anyone else, including the GP and family (**IV, C**).

iii A plan should be made for the management of the individual and for the further investigation of the family (**IV, C**).

iv *The individual.* Mutation implies MEN2 and thus (depending on the site of the mutation) a future risk of other MEN2 components such as further thyroid tumours, adrenal and parathyroid disease.

v   *The family.* Family members at risk should be offered testing for the specific *RET* mutation (**IV, C**).

vi Contacting and investigating the family require expertise and co-ordination and should normally be undertaken by a specialist clinical genetics department, in liaison with the relevant clinical teams (**IV, C**).

If no mutation is found

i   Check with the genetics laboratory that a complete mutation screen has been carried out, to include exons 10, 11 and 13–16 of the *RET* gene. If not, ask for this to be completed (IV, C).

ii   If there is strong presumptive evidence from the individual or family history of inherited disease:

   (a) discuss further with the clinical genetics department and consider research-based search for novel mutations (IV, C)

   (b) consider biochemical screening of family members at risk using stimulated (intravenous calcium/pentagastrin, Appendix 1) calcitonin testing from age 5 years.

iii If there is no clinical evidence to suggest inherited disease, the need for stimulated calcitonin screening of family members at risk is unclear. There are a few MEN2 families (mostly with FMTC only) in which *RET* mutations have not so far been identified. Thus, a failure to find a *RET* mutation in an isolated case of MTC cannot completely exclude the possibility of heritable disease. The extent of the remaining risk is very small – around 1% or less, depending on the clinical features of the patient. Young age at onset of the MTC (<35 years) and the presence of CCH in the thyroid are suggestive of inherited disease, but not conclusive, nor does the absence of these features exclude it. The correct action in this situation is a matter for clinical judgement and may differ from family to family.

Mutation testing of tumour

i   If no blood sample is available from the affected individual, DNA may be obtainable from either frozen or paraffin-embedded tumour.

ii   Interpretation of *RET* mutations identified from tumour tissue requires care. The mutations may be either germline or somatic in origin. Specialist genetic advice should be sought (IV, C).

iii A somatic MEN2B-type (codon 918) mutation is commonly present in sporadic tumours, but may also be present in tumours from MEN2A cases. This finding cannot therefore be used to exclude heritable disease.

14.7 Multiple endocrine neoplasia 2B (MEN2B)

Recognition

Photographs to aid diagnosis are provided in Appendix 2. MTC occurs early in MEN2B and is particularly aggressive.[212,249]

i   Any new patient with MTC, especially a child or young adult, should be carefully assessed for clinical features suggestive of MEN2B[198,210,250,251] (III, B).

ii   The clinical features of MEN2B may be hard to recognise and the syndrome is sometimes diagnosed in error.

iii More than 98% of MEN2B patients reported to date have mutations in either *RET* codon 918 (95%) or 883 (3%). Unless the clinical evidence is strong, preferably with radiological and/or biopsy support, the absence of these mutations excludes MEN2B with high probability. Where there is doubt, the patient should be referred for a specialist opinion[251,252] (IV, C).

Child of an MEN2B patient

i   Because MEN2B can present with clinically significant MTC in the neonatal period, management of the newborn child of a known MEN2B carrier should be planned in advance with specialist advice **(IV, C)**.

ii   Because MTC occurs early in MEN2B and is particularly aggressive, thyroid surgery in an affected child should be done as early as possible, preferably before the age of 12 months[221] **(III, B)**.

iii   Prenatal testing is possible. Couples who ask about prenatal testing for MEN2 should be referred to a genetics clinic **(IV, C)**.

15 Registration, core dataset and audit

It is mandatory for all patients with thyroid cancer in England and Wales to be registered within a regional cancer network. Further information on the core dataset can be found on: **www.ic.nhs.uk**

Prospective data collection and regular audit of outcomes and processes should be carried out (**IV, C**).

The primary purpose is to ensure that all patients are adequately followed up.

The development of a national dataset will allow audit of national outcomes and provide the potential for prospective assessment of different treatment modalities. This comprises a thyroid cancer-specific dataset which has been in use at one hospital for the past decade and has undergone serial modifications during that time. This could be implemented for general use immediately to record treatment and relapse, and to facilitate audit. Subsequent analysis would then permit improvements in treatment and also setting up of prospective clinical trials. The Information Centre for Health and Social Care is developing a generic dataset for all cancers; this is available on **www.ic.nhs.uk**

The proformas should be completed by a member of the MDT (**IV, C**).

16 Thyroid cancer: a guide for general practitioners

16.1 Raising awareness

i   Thyroid nodules, particularly when solitary and clinically obvious, should be investigated as they carry a small but significant malignant potential (about 10% or less).

ii Cancer of the thyroid is rare, representing only about 1% of all cancers.

iii The overall 10-year survival rate for DTC is 80–90%.

iv 5–20% of patients develop local or regional recurrences and 10–15% develop distant metastases.

16.2 Prevention

i   Previous head or neck irradiation in childhood is a possible cause of thyroid cancer in adults. Exposure to radiation should be limited whenever possible.

ii Nuclear fallout is a well recognised cause of increased risk of thyroid cancer.

iii If populations or individuals are contaminated with radioactive iodine, the thyroid can be protected by administering potassium iodide.[254,255]

16.3 Screening

No screening is indicated for the general population.

Risk-directed screening should be considered (by referral to the specialist secondary team) when the GP identifies patients with:

- familial thyroid cancer, including MTC
- history of neck irradiation in childhood
- family history of MEN2.

Patients with the following carry a statistically increased risk of thyroid malignancy but no screening is recommended:

- endemic goitre
- Hashimoto's thyroiditis (risk of lymphoma)
- family or personal history of thyroid adenoma
- Cowden's syndrome (macrocephaly, mild learning difficulties, carpet-pile tongue, with benign or malignant breast disease)
- familial adenomatous polyposis.

16.4 Diagnosis and referral

The usual presentation is that of a palpable lump in the neck, which moves on swallowing. There may be no other symptoms or signs.

Immediate (same day) referrals

Patients with stridor associated with a thyroid swelling should be referred immediately to secondary care. (Depending on locally provided facilities, this may be the accident and emergency department, head and neck or general surgical emergency services.)

Urgent referrals under the 2-week rule for suspected cancer

The presence of the following symptoms or signs in association with a thyroid swelling may indicate more aggressive or advanced disease and should be referred urgently under the 2-week rule:

- unexplained hoarseness or voice change
- thyroid nodule/goitre in a child
- cervical lymphadenopathy associated with a thyroid lump (usually deep cervical or supraclavicular region)
- a rapidly enlarging painless thyroid mass over a period of weeks (a rare presentation of thyroid cancer and usually associated with anaplastic thyroid cancer or thyroid lymphoma).

Patients in whom exclusion of thyroid cancer is required should be referred to a thyroid nodule clinic, or a surgeon, endocrinologist or nuclear medicine physician who has a special interest in thyroid cancer and is a member of the regional thyroid cancer MDT.

Non-urgent referrals

The following patients should be referred in the normal way:

- patients with nodules who have abnormal TFTs, who should be referred to an endocrinologist (thyroid cancer is very rare in this group)
- patients with a history of sudden onset of pain in a thyroid lump (likely to have bled into a benign thyroid cyst)_
- patients with a thyroid lump that is newly presenting or has been increasing in size over months.

Physical examination

i   Examination should focus on inspection and palpation of the thyroid and neck, movement of the nodule with swallowing, and palpation of the deep cervical nodes and all other node groups in the neck especially supraclavicular nodes.

ii Pulse and blood pressure should be noted.

Appropriate investigations pending hospital appointment

i   Thyroid function tests should be requested by the GP and appended to the referral letter. Hyperthyroidism or hypothyroidism associated with a nodular goitre is unlikely to be thyroid cancer; these patients should be referred routinely to an endocrinologist.

ii Initiation of other investigations (such as ultrasound scanning or autoantibodies) by the GP is unnecessary and may cause delay in making the diagnosis of cancer.

The diagnosis and management of a thyroid nodule or suspected thyroid cancer in general practice is presented in schematic form in Fig 2.

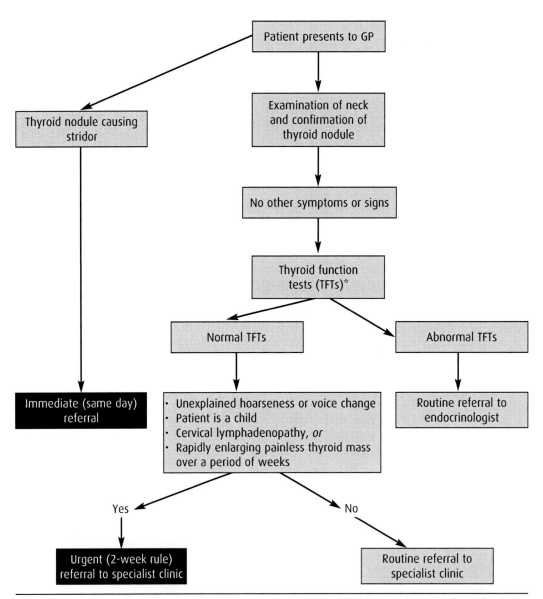

Fig 2. Algorithm for the diagnosis and management of a thyroid nodule or suspected thyroid cancer in general practice.

* There is no need to arrange ultrasound of thyroid.

Communicating the diagnosis

Informing the primary care team

i The GP should expect to be informed within 24 hours (by telephone or fax) of the diagnosis of thyroid cancer being communicated to the patient for the first time and should be made aware of the information which has been given to the patient and of the planned treatment.

ii Subsequent alterations in prognosis, management or drug treatment should be communicated promptly.

Informing the patient

i The patient should be informed of the diagnosis by a member of the specialist team.

ii A trained nurse specialist should be available in the specialist clinic to provide additional counselling if required.

iii Whenever possible a relative or friend should attend the hospital consultation and accompany the patient home.

iv Written information concerning thyroid cancer and its treatment should be available to the patient in the specialist clinic.

v A prognosis will not be offered before adequate staging information is available.

vi Patients may have difficulty understanding all this information at a single consultation and an opportunity for further explanation/discussion will be offered.

16.5 Summary of treatment of thyroid cancer

Treatment decisions will be made by the thyroid cancer MDT who will continue to supervise the patient's care.

i Patients will commonly undergo thyroidectomy, followed in some cases by an ablative dose of radioiodine (^{131}I).

ii Thereafter patients will generally require thyroxine to suppress TSH to <0.1 miu/L and some will need treatment to correct hypocalcaemia.

iii Scans and/or measurement of Tg will be performed at regular intervals to detect possible recurrence.

iv Patients will be provided with written and verbal information about the disease and its management.

v Pregnancy: radioiodine is not given to pregnant patients. Pregnancy must be avoided for six months after ^{131}I ablation or therapy in women and 4 months in men. Breastfeeding needs to be stopped at least 4 weeks and preferably 8 weeks before radioiodine ablation or therapy and not be resumed.

16.6 Follow-up

Follow-up of patients with thyroid cancer is lifelong and usually supervised by specialists in secondary or tertiary care who are members of the MDT. Low-risk cases who have completed their treatment, are shown to be free of disease at 5 years and no longer judged to require TSH suppression, may be followed up in settings other than the multidisciplinary thyroid cancer clinic. This may be a nurse-led clinic or in primary care following agreement of well defined

protocols and re-referral pathways.

i   *Thyroxine treatment:* The dose of levothyroxine is usually higher than a normal replacement dose as it is intended to suppress the level of serum TSH to undetectable. For example, if the TSH is in the normal range, the dose of levothyroxine will usually be *increased.* Suppressive levothyroxine therapy is best supervised by a member of the thyroid cancer MDT, preferably an endocrinologist. The GP will be advised of the target levels of TSH.

ii   *Treatment of hypocalcaemia:* Patients taking calcitriol/alfacalcidol and/or calcium supplements must be monitored closely (eg every 3 months until stable, annually thereafter) to ensure that hypercalcaemia does not occur. The dose is kept to the minimum required to maintain serum calcium in the (low) normal range.

iii   The GP should ensure that the patient knows about and is offered:

- *MDT follow-up* – necessary for detection of early recurrence and complications and for their appropriate treatment
- access to a member of the core team for support.

Appendix 1 Assay methodology

1 Measurement of thyroglobulin

Many differentiated papillary and follicular carcinomas of the thyroid synthesise and secrete Tg. Detailed UK guidelines for measurements of relevant analytes have been published[55] and will be summarised here. Problems with Tg assays have been widely reviewed.[55,124,156,157,256–258]

i   There should be clear guidance from each laboratory to its users on specimen requirements and sample stability (**IV, C**).

ii The use of the Community Bureau of Reference standard for Tg (CRM 457) is recommended (**IV, C**).

iii The use of a reference range derived from normal subjects is not recommended. The laboratory should ensure that users are aware that patients on levothyroxine suppressive therapy should ideally have an undetectable serum Tg[55] (**IV, C**).

iv Laboratories and manufacturers should determine and quote the minimum detection limit (MDL) of their assay based on functional sensitivity derived from patient samples. The MDL should ideally be ≤0.2 µg/L (**IV, C**).

v   Although a post-rhTSH serum Tg of ≥2 µg/L has been suggested as a positive response justifying further investigations and treatment, this threshold may not be applicable for many of the currently available assays because of known differences in sensitivity, accuracy and precision (**IV, C**).

vi Laboratories and manufacturers should identify the analytical range of their Tg assay and adopt procedures to identify samples suffering from 'hook' effects (**IV, C**).

vii Laboratories and manufacturers should inform clinicians of the possibility of interference due to endogenous TgAb and indicate the most likely nature of the interference (false elevation/false reduction in measured Tg) (**IV, C**).

viii Identification of possible assay interference is best achieved using either TgAb measurements or discordance between Tg results obtained using immunometric assay and radioimmunoassay (RIA).[258] Recovery experiments alone are not recommended to identify assay interference[256] (**IV, C**). In the presence of antibody interference RIAs perform better than immunometric assays. In such cases, measurement of serum Tg by RIA may be helpful.

ix TgAb should be measured in the same sample as serum Tg. The presence of TgAb usually invalidates the serum Tg result but interference may also occur in the absence of TgAb. If TgAb are to be measured a sensitive immunoassay rather than a haemaglutination method should be used[55] (**IV, C**).

x   For a particular Tg method it is highly desirable that the results of a clinical assessment of the assay performance should be available. The clinical sensitivity and specificity (ie positive and negative predictive values) of the assays should be quoted (**IV, C**).

xi Laboratories should run internal quality control samples, which encompass the range of results reported by the laboratory. A sample with a Tg concentration close to the MDL should also be run with each assay to ensure that the quoted MDL is being achieved (**IV, C**).

xii Laboratories should participate in an accredited external quality assessment scheme (IV, C).

xiii Requesting clinicians should contact the laboratory before the collection of blood for Tg/TSH from patients post-radioiodine administration (IV, C). The handling and transport of such radioactive samples are covered by legislation and such samples may not be accepted by the laboratory.

2 Measurement of calcitonin

The following recommendations apply to the measurement of calcitonin (IV, C).

Timing of specimen collection

i   Ideally a fasting morning specimen should be obtained to enable optimal comparison with reference values. If this is not possible, specimens can be collected at any time of day.

ii Postoperative samples should be collected no earlier than 10 days after thyroidectomy and should also be fasting samples if possible[55,224] (III, B).

iii For provocative testing, samples are usually collected 5 minutes prior to administration of calcium/pentagastrin and then at intervals of 2, 5 and 7–10 minutes after.[156] Indications for provocative testing are listed in 14.2iv.

Type of specimen

i   Serum or plasma requirements should be confirmed with laboratories and/or manufacturers' kit inserts. The effect of gel tubes should be known (IV, C).

ii Calcitonin results may be affected by visible haemolysis or lipaemia and assay of such specimens should be avoided if possible.

Specimen stability

Calcitonin in serum or plasma is unstable and blood specimens should be kept on ice. Red cells should then be separated within 30 minutes of collection and serum or plasma frozen immediately (IV, C).

Effects of other conditions, treatment and medication

i   Previous treatment with monoclonal antibodies should be noted because of the potential for interference with human anti-mouse antibodies in immunometric assays (IV, C).

ii Chronic renal failure may increase basal calcitonin levels.

iii Mildly increased calcitonin may be observed in pregnancy, pernicious anaemia, autoimmune thyroid disease, hypergastrinaemia and during the neonatal period.

Methodology

i   Assays should be standardised using WHO International Standard IS 89/620 (IV, C).

ii Laboratories must decide whether to use a method that recognises primarily monomeric calcitonin (immunometric) or a method with broader specificity (RIA) (IV, C).

Assay sensitivity

Laboratories and/or manufacturers should determine and quote the MDL of their assay based on precision profiles derived from patient samples (IV, C).

Assay interferences

Laboratories should have established protocols for identifying specimens that may have 'hooked' and those that may contain interfering antibodies (IV, C).

Clinical assessment

For a particular calcitonin method the results of a clinical assessment of the assay performance should be available. The clinical sensitivity and specificity (ie positive and negative predictive values) of the assays should be quoted.

Quality assurance

i   Laboratories should run internal quality control at concentrations appropriate for the range of results obtained. A pool with a calcitonin concentration close to the minimum detectable limit should also be run to ensure good baseline security (IV, C).

ii Laboratories should participate in a recognised and accredited external quality assessment scheme (IV, C).

Appendix 2 Recognition of MEN2B

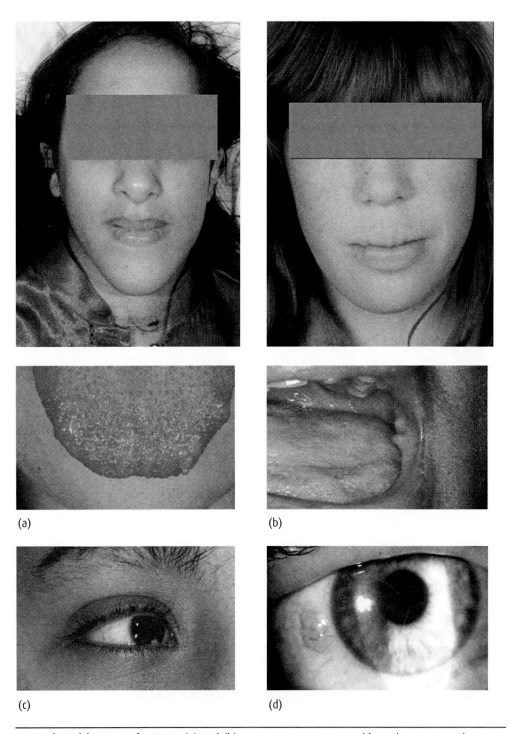

(a)

(b)

(c)

(d)

Fig 3. Clinical features of MEN2B. (a) and (b) neuromas on tongue and buccal mucosa, and irregular dentition and high arch palate; (c) and (d) neuromas on eyelid, and conjunctival neuromas and thickened corneal nerves on slit-lamp examination. (Reproduced with the consent of the patients.)

Appendix 3 Search methodology

Literature searches were carried out on a number of databases and worldwide web resources. There are few systematic reviews and randomised controlled trials in this area so a search strategy was designed to retrieve reviews and papers reporting on all primary studies including cohort studies, case-control studies and other clinical trials. No limit was placed on language or age of subjects or on date of publication.

It was also necessary to limit searches to DTC, and exclude undifferentiated anaplastic thyroid cancer. The search therefore included the following items:

> DTC
>
> Thyroid neoplasm
>
> Thyroid nodule
>
> Carcinoma – papillary, follicular
>
> Oncocytic follicular (Hürthle cell) carcinomas
>
> MTC
>
> MEN2.

A medline search covered 1966–2006.

This was supplemented by searches on the Cochrane Library and a number of worldwide web resources, including:

> Cancerlit
>
> CancerNet
>
> National Guideline Clearinghouse
>
> National Research Register
>
> Scottish Intercollegiate Guidelines Network (SIGN).

Appendix 4 References

1   National Institute for Clinical Excellence. *Guidance on cancer services – improving outcomes in head and neck cancers.* London: NICE, 2004. www.nice.org.uk/pdf/csghn_themanual.pdf

2   Spoudeas HA (ed). *Paediatric endocrine tumours. A multi-disciplinary consensus statement of best practice from a working group convened under the auspices of the BSPED and UKCCSG.* Crawley: Novo Nordisk, 2005.

3   Agency for Health Care Policy and Research. *Acute pain management: operative or medical procedures and trauma.* Clinical practice guideline number 1. Rockville, MD: AHCPR, 1992:107.

4   Agency for Health Care Policy and Research. *Management of cancer pain: adults.* Clinical practice guideline number 9. Rockville, MD: AHCPR, 1994.

5   Department of Health. www.dh.gov.uk/en/policyandguidance/healthandsocialcaretopics/cancer/dh4135595

6   Teppo L, Hakulinen T. Variation in survival of adult patients with thyroid cancer in Europe. *Eur J Cancer* 1998;34:2248–52.

7   Coleman PM, Babb P, Damiecki P *et al. Cancer survival trends in England and Wales 1971–1995: deprivation and NHS region.* Series SMPS No. 61. London: Stationery Office, 1999:471–8.

8   Toms JR (ed). *CancerStats monograph 2004. Cancer incidence, survival and mortality in the UK and EU.* London: Cancer Research UK, 2004.

9   Mazzaferri EL. An overview of the management of papillary and follicular thyroid carcinoma. *Thyroid* 1999;9:421–7.

10 Loh KC, Greenspan FS, Gee L, Miller TR, Yeo PP. Pathological tumor-node-metastasis (pTNM) staging for papillary and follicular thyroid carcinomas: a retrospective analysis of 700 patients. *J Clin Endocrinol Metab* 1997;82:3553–62.

11 D'Avanzo A, Ituarte P, Treseler P *et al.* Prognostic scoring systems in patients with follicular thyroid cancer: a comparison of different staging systems in predicting the patient outcome. *Thyroid* 2004;14:453–8.

12 Wittekind C, Meyer H, Bootz F (eds). *TNM. Klassifikation maligner Tumoren,* 5th edn. Berlin: Springer, 1997.

12a Brierley JD, Panzarella T. A comparison of different staging systems predictability of patient outcome. Thyroid carcinoma as an example. *Cancer* 1997;79:2414–23.

12b Passler C, Prager G, Scheuba C *et al.* Application of staging systems for differentiated thyroid carcinoma in an endemic goiter region with iodine substitution. *Ann Surg* 2003;237:227–34.

12c Lo CY, Chan WF, Lam KY, Wan KY. Follicular thyroid carcinoma: the role of histology and staging systems in predicting survival. *Ann Surg* 2005;242:708–15.

13 Mazzaferri EL, Jhiang SM. Long-term impact of initial surgical and medical therapy on papillary and follicular thyroid cancer. *Am J Med* 1994;97:418–28.

14 Carcangiu ML, Zampi G, Pupi A, Castagnoli A, Rosai J. Papillary carcinoma of the thyroid. A clinicopathologic study of 241 cases treated at the University of Florence, Italy. *Cancer* 1985;55:805–28.

15 Simpson WJ, McKinney SE, Carruthers JS *et al.* Papillary and follicular thyroid cancer: prognostic factors in 1578 patients. *Am J Med* 1987;83:479–88.

16 Tubiana M, Schlumberger M, Rougier P *et al.* Long-term results and prognostic factors in patients with differentiated thyroid carcinoma. *Cancer* 1985;55:794–804.

17 Akslen LA, Haldorsen T, Thoresen SO, Glattre E. Survival and causes of death in thyroid cancer: a population-based study of 2479 cases from Norway. *Cancer Res* 1991;51:1234–41.

18 Hay ID. Papillary thyroid carcinoma. *Endocrinol Metab Clin North Am* 1990;19:545–76.

19 Furmanchuk AW, Averkin JI, Egloff B *et al.* Pathomorphological findings in thyroid cancers of children from the Republic of Belarus: a study of 86 cases occurring between 1986 ('post-Chernobyl') and 1991. *Histopathology* 1992;21:401–8.

20 Schlumberger M, De Vathaire F, Travagli JP *et al.* Differentiated thyroid carcinoma in childhood: long term follow-up of 72 patients. *J Clin Endocrinol Metab* 1987;65:1088–94.

21 Cady B, Rossi R. An expanded view of risk group definition in differentiated thyroid carcinoma. *Surgery* 1988;104:947–53.

22 Brennan M, Bergstralh EH, Heerden JA, McConahey WM. Follicular thyroid cancer treated at the Mayo Clinic 1946–1970. Initial manifestation, pathologic findings, therapy and outcome. *Mayo Clinic Proc* 1991;66:11–22.

23 Emerick GT, Duh QY, Siperstein AE *et al.* Diagnosis, treatment and outcome of follicular thyroid carcinoma. *Cancer* 1993;72:3287–95.

24   Donohue JH, Goldfien SD, Miller TR, Abele JS, Clark OH. Do the prognoses of papillary and follicular thyroid carcinomas differ? *Am J Surg* 1984;148:168–73.

25   Evans HL. Columnar-cell carcinoma of the thyroid. A report of two cases of an aggressive variant of thyroid carcinoma. *Am J Clin Pathol* 1986;85:77–80.

26   Herrera MF, Hay ID, Wu PS *et al*. Hurthle cell (oxyphilic) papillary thyroid carcinoma: a variant with more aggressive biologic behavior. *World J Surg* 1992;16:669–74.

27   Akslen LA, LiVolsi VA. Prognostic significance of histologic grading compared with subclassification of papillary thyroid carcinoma. *Cancer* 2000;88:1902.

28   Rosai J, Zampi G, Carcangiu ML. Papillary carcinoma of the thyroid. A discussion of its several morphologic expressions, with particular emphasis on the follicular variant. *Am J Surg Pathol* 1983;7:809–17.

29   Hay ID, Bergstralh EJ, Goellner JR, Ebersold JR, Grant CS. Predicting outcome in papillary thyroid carcinoma: Development of a reliable prognostic scoring system in a cohort of 1779 patients surgically treated at one institution during 1940 through 1989. *Surgery* 1993;114:1050–8.

30   Lang W, Choritz H, Hundeshagen H. Risk factors in follicular thyroid carcinomas. A retrospective follow-up study covering a 14-year period with emphasis on morphological findings. *Am J Surg Pathol* 1986;10:246–55.

31   DeGroot LJ, Kaplan EL, Shukla MS, Salti G, Straus FH. Morbidity and mortality in follicular thyroid cancer. *J Clin Endocrinol Metab* 1995;80:2946–53.

32   Yamashita H, Noguchi S, Murakami N, Kawamoto H, Watanabe S. Extracapsular invasion of lymph node metastasis is an indicator of distant metastasis and poor prognosis in patients with thyroid papillary carcinoma. *Cancer* 1997;80:2268–72.

33   DeGroot LJ, Kaplan EL, McCormick M, Straus FH. Natural history, treatment and course of papillary thyroid cancer. *J Clin Endocrinol Metab* 1990;71:414–24.

34   Dinneen SF, Valimaki MJ, Bergstralh EJ *et al*. Distant metastases in papillary thyroid carcinoma: 100 cases observed at one institution during 5 decades. *J Clin Endocrinol Metab* 1995;80: 2041–5.

35   Hoie J, Stenwig AE, Kullmann G, Lindegaard M. Distant metastases in papillary thyroid cancer. A review of 91 patients. *Cancer* 1988;61:1–6.

36   Pacini F, Cetani F, Miccoli P *et al*. Outcome of 309 patients with metastatic differentiated thyroid carcinoma treated with radioiodine. *World J Surg* 1994;18:600–4.

36a   Administration of Radioactive Substances Advisory Committee. *Notes for guidance on the clinical administration of radiopharmaceuticals and use of sealed radioactive sources.* Didcot, Oxon: ARSAC, 2006. www.arsac.org.uk/notes_for_guidence/index.htm

37   International Atomic Energy Agency. *Intervention criteria in a nuclear or nuclear radiation emergency.* Safety series number 109. Vienna: IAEA, 1991.

38   International Commission on Radiological Protection. *ICRP publication 63: Principles for intervention for protection of the public in radiological emergency.* Oxford: Pergamon Press, 1991.

39   Giordano TJ, Kuick R, Thomas DG *et al*. Molecular classification of papillary thyroid carcinoma: distinct BRAF, RAS, and RET/PTC mutation-specific gene expression profiles discovered by DNA microarray analysis. *Oncogene* 2005;24:6646–56.

40   Hancock SL, Cox RS, McDougall IR. Thyroid disease after treatment of Hodgkin's disease. *N Engl J Med* 1991;325:599–605.

41   Ron E, Lubin JH, Shore RE *et al*. Thyroid cancer after exposure of external radiation: a pooled analysis of seven studies. *Radiat Res* 1995;141:259–77.

42   Thompson DE, Mabuchi K, Ron E *et al*. Cancer incidence in atomic bomb survivors. Part II: Solid tumors, 1958–1987. *Radiat Res* 1994;137(2 Suppl):S17–67.

43   Winship T, Rosvoll RV. Thyroid carcinoma in childhood: final report on a 20 year study. *Clin Proc Child Hosp Dis* 1970;26:327–48.

44   Franceschi S, Boyle P, Maisonneuve P *et al*. The epidemiology of thyroid carcinoma. *Crit Rev Oncogen* 1993;4:25–52.

45   Levi F, Franceschi S, la Vecchia C *et al*. Prior thyroid disease and risk of thyroid cancer in Switzerland. *Eur J Cancer* 1991;27:85–8.

46   Preston-Martin S, Berenstein L, Pike MC, Maldonado AA, Henderson BE. Thyroid cancer among young women related to prior thyroid disease and pregnancy history. *Br J Cancer* 1987;55:191–5.

47   Mack WJ, Preston-Martin S. Epidemiology of thyroid cancer. In: Fagin JA (ed). *Thyroid cancer*, vol 2. Boston: Kluwer Academic Publishers, 1998:1–25.

48   Holm LE, Blomgren H, Lowhagen T. Cancer risks in patients with chronic lymphocytic thyroiditis. *N Engl J Med* 1985;312:601–4.

49   Hegedus L. Clinical practice. The thyroid nodule. *N Engl J Med* 2004;351:1764–71.

50   Department of Health. *Cancer waiting times: a guide* (version 5). London: DH, 2006. www.dh.gov.uk/en/Publicationsandstatistics/Publications/PublicationsPolicyAndGuidance/DH_063067

51 Department of Health. *Manual of cancer services assessment standards, consultation document.* London: DH, 2000. http://www.dh.gov.uk/en/Publicationsandstatistics/Publications/PublicationsPolicyAndGuidance/DH_063067

52 Kumar H, Daykin J, Holder R *et al.* Gender, clinical findings and serum thyrotropin measurements in the prediction of thyroid neoplasia in 1005 patients presenting with thyroid enlargement and investigated by fine needle aspiration cytology (FNAC). *Thyroid* 1999;9:1105–9.

53 Cap J, Ryska A, Rehorkova P *et al.* Sensitivity and specificity of the fine needle aspiration biopsy of the thyroid: clinical point of view. *Clin Endocrinol* 1999;51:509–15.

54 Danese D, Sciacchitano S, Farsetti A *et al.* Diagnostic accuracy of conventional versus sonography-guided fine-needle aspiration biopsy of thyroid nodules. *Thyroid* 1998;8:15–21.

54a Baskin HJ. Ultrasound-guided fine-needle aspiration biopsy of thyroid nodules and multinodular goiters. *Endocr Pract* 2004;10:242–5.

55 Association of Clinical Biochemistry, British Thyroid Association, British Thyroid Foundation. *UK guidelines for the use of thyroid function tests.* London: ACB, 2006. www.acb.org.uk/docs/TFTguidelinefinal.pdf#search=%22propylthiouracil%20manufacturer%20uk%22

56 Elisei R, Bottici V, Luchetti F *et al.* Impact of routine measurement of serum calcitonin on the diagnosis and outcome of medullary thyroid cancer: experience in 10,864 patients with nodular thyroid disorders. *J Clin Endocrinol Metab* 2004;89:163–8.

57 Rieu M, Lame MC, Richard A *et al.* Prevalence of sporadic medullary thyroid carcinoma: the importance of routine measurement of serum calcitonin in the diagnostic evaluation of thyroid nodules. *Clin Endocrinol* 1995;42:453–60.

58 Gittoes NJ, Miller MR, Daykin J, Sheppard MC, Franklyn JA. Upper airways obstruction in 153 consecutive patients presenting with thyroid enlargement. *BMJ* 1996;312:484.

59 Rojeski MT, Gharib H. Nodular thyroid disease: evaluation and management. *N Engl J Med* 1985;313:428–36.

60 Giuffrida D, Gharib H. Controversies in the management of cold, hot and occult thyroid nodules. *Am J Med* 1995;99:642–50.

61 Tabaqchali MA, Hanson JM, Johnson SJ *et al.* Thyroid aspiration cytology in Newcastle: a six year cytology/histology correlation study. *Ann R Coll Surg Engl* 2000;82:149–55.

62 Sclabas GM, Staerkel GA, Shapiro SE *et al.* Fine-needle aspiration of the thyroid and correlation with histopathology in a contemporary series of 240 patients. *Am J Surg* 2003;186:702–9.

63 Caron NR, Cord S, Clark OH. The specialist endocrine surgeon. In: Mazzaferri EL, Harmer C, Mallick UK, Kendall-Taylor P (eds). *Practical management of thyroid cancer: a multidisciplinary approach.* London: Springer, 2006:121–34.

64 Mallick UK. Thyroid cancer multidisciplinary team and the organisational paradigm. In: Mazzaferri EL, Harmer C, Mallick UK, Kendall-Taylor P (eds) *Practical management of thyroid cancer: a multidisciplinary approach.* London: Springer, 2006:39–53.

65 Department of Health. *Head and neck specific measures.* London: DH, 2004. www.dh.gov.uk/assetRoot/04/13/55/91/04135591.pdf

65a Wells PS, Lensing AW, Hirsh J. Graduated compression stockings in the prevention of postoperative venous thromboembolism. A meta-analysis. *Arch Intern Med* 1994;154:67–72.

66 Randolph GW. The importance of preoperative laryngoscopy in patients undergoing thyroidectomy: voice, vocal cord function, and the preoperative detection of invasive thyroid malignancy. *Surgery* 2006;139:363–4.

67 Watkinson JC, Franklyn JA, Olliff JF. Detection and surgical treatment of cervical lymph nodes in differentiated thyroid cancer. *Thyroid* 2006;16:187–94.

68 Schlumberger MJ. Papillary and follicular thyroid carcinoma. *N Engl J Med* 1998;338:297–306.

69 Cooper DS, Doherty GM, Haugen BR *et al.* The American Thyroid Association Guidelines Taskforce. Management guidelines for patients with thyroid nodules and differentiated thyroid cancer. *Thyroid* 2006;16:109–42.

70 Pacini F, Schlumberger M, Dralle H *et al.* European Thyroid Cancer Taskforce. European consensus for the management of patients with differentiated thyroid carcinoma of the follicular epithelium. *Eur J Endocrinol* 2006;154:787–803.

71 Bi J, Lu B. Advances in diagnosis and management of thyroid neoplasms. *Curr Opin Oncol* 2000;12:54–9.

72 Hundahl SA, Cady B, Cunningham MP *et al.* Initial results from a prospective cohort study of 5583 cases of thyroid carcinoma treated in the United States during 1996. US and German Thyroid Cancer Study Group. An American College of Surgeons Cancer Patient Care Evaluation Study. *Cancer* 2000;89:202–17.

73 Van De Velde CJ, Hamming JF, Goslings BM *et al.* Report of the consensus development conference on the management of differentiated thyroid cancer in the Netherlands. *Eur J Cancer* 1988;24:287–92.

74 Falk SA, McCaffrey TV. Management of recurrent laryngeal nerve in suspected and proven thyroid cancer. *Otolaryngol Head Neck Surg* 1995;113:42–8.

75 Cernea CR, Ferraz AR, Monteiro S *et al.* Identification of the external branch of the superior laryngeal nerve during thyroidectomy. *Am J Surg* 1992;164:634–9.

76 Lennquist S, Cahlin C, Smeds S. The superior laryngeal nerve in thyroid surgery. *Surgery* 1987;102:999–1008.

77 Olson JA Jr, DeBenedetti MK, Baumann DS, Wells SA Jr. Parathyroid autotransplantation during thyroidectomy. Results of long-term follow-up. *Ann Surg* 1996;223:472–80.

78 Cheah WK, Arici C, Ituarte PH *et al.* Complications of neck dissection for thyroid cancer. *World J Surg* 2002;26:1013–6.

79 van Santen HM, Aronson DC, Vulsma T *et al.* Frequent adverse events after treatment for childhood-onset differentiated thyroid carcinoma: a single institute experience. *Eur J Cancer* 2004;40:1743–51.

80 Dralle H, Damm I, Scheumann GF *et al.* Compartment-oriented microdissection of regional nodes in medullary thyroid carcinoma. *Surg Today* 1994;24:112–21.

81 Mulcahy MM, Cohen JI, Anderson PE, Ditamasso J, Schmidt W. Relative accuracy of fine-needle aspiration and frozen section in the diagnosis of well-differentiated thyroid cancer. *Laryngoscope* 1998;104:494–6.

82 van Heerden JA, Hay ID, Goellner RJ *et al.* Follicular thyroid carcinoma with capsular invasion alone: a non threatening malignancy. *Surgery* 1992;112:1130–6.

83 Pacini F, Schlumberger M, Harmer C *et al.* Post-surgical use of radioiodine (131I) in patients with papillary and follicular thyroid cancer and the issue of remnant ablation: a consensus report. *Eur J Endocrinol* 2005;153:651–9.

84 Sobrinho-Simoes M, Maximo V, Castro IV *et al.* Hurthle (oncocytic) cell tumors of thyroid: etiopathogenesis, diagnosis and clinical significance. *Int J Surg Pathol* 2005;13:29–35.

85 Pearce EN, Braverman LE. Papillary thyroid microcarcinoma outcomes and implications for treatment. *J Clin Endocrinol Metab* 2004;89:3710–2.

86 Drucker WD, Robbins RJ. Papillary microcarcinoma. In: Mazzaferri EL, Harmer C, Mallick UK, Kendall-Taylor P (eds). *Practical management of thyroid cancer: a multidisciplinary approach.* London: Springer, 2006:371–89.

87 Mazzaferri EL. An overview of the management of thyroid cancer. In: Mazzaferri EL, Harmer C, Mallick UK, Kendall-Taylor P (eds). *Practical management of thyroid cancer: a multidisciplinary approach.* London: Springer, 2006:1–28.

88 Feldt-Rasmussen U, Petersen PH, Date J, Madsen CM. Serum thyroglobulin in patients undergoing subtotal thyroidectomy for toxic and nontoxic goiter. *J Endocrinol Invest* 1982;5:161–4.

89 Izumi M, Kubo I, Taura M *et al.* Kinetic study of immunoreactive human thyroglobulin. *J Clin Endocrinol Metab* 1986;62:410–2.

90 Ozata M, Suzuki S, Miyamoto T *et al.* Serum thyroglobulin in the follow-up of patients with treated differentiated thyroid cancer. *J Clin Endocrinol Metab* 1994;79:98–105.

91 Hocevar M, Auersperg M, Stanovnik L. The dynamics of serum thyroglobulin elimination from the body after thyroid surgery. *Eur J Surg Oncol* 1997;23:208–10.

92 Cha C, Chen H, Westra WH, Udelsman R. Primary thyroid lymphoma: can the diagnosis be made solely by fine-needle aspiration? *Ann Surg Oncol* 2002;9:298–302.

93 Harrington KJ, Michalaki VJ, Vini L *et al.* Management of non-Hodgkin's lymphoma of the thyroid: the Royal Marsden Hospital experience. *Br J Radiol* 2005;78:405–10.

94 Giuffrida D, Gharib H. Anaplastic thyroid carcinoma: current diagnosis and treatment. *Ann Oncol* 2000;11:1083–9.

95 Haigh PI, Ituarte PH, Wu HS *et al.* Completely resected anaplastic thyroid carcinoma combined with adjuvant chemotherapy and irradiation is associated with prolonged survival. *Cancer* 2001;91:2335–42.

96 Haq M, Harmer C. Non-surgical management of thyroid cancer. In: Mazzaferri EL, Harmer C, Mallick UK, Kendall-Taylor P (eds). *Practical management of thyroid cancer: a multidisciplinary approach.* London: Springer, 2006:171–91.

97 Pluijmen MJ, Eustatia-Rutten C, Goslings BM *et al.* Effects of low-iodide diet on postsurgical radioiodide ablation therapy in patients with differentiated thyroid carcinoma. *Clin Endocrinol* 2003;58:428–35.

98 Lakshmanan M, Schaffer A, Robbins J, Reynolds J, Norton J. A simplified low iodine diet in I-131 scanning and therapy of thyroid cancer. *Clin Nucl Med* 1988;13:866–8.

99 Maxon HR. Quantitative radioiodine therapy in the treatment of differentiated thyroid cancer. *Q J Nucl Med* 1999;43:313–23.

100 Maxon HR, Smith HS. Radioiodine-131 in the diagnosis and treatment of metastatic well differentiated thyroid cancer. *Endocrinol Metab Clin North Am* 1990;19:685–718.

101 Leger F A, Izembart M, Dagousset F *et al.* Decreased uptake of therapeutic doses of iodine 131 after 185-MBq iodine-131 diagnostic imaging for thyroid remnants in differentiated thyroid carcinoma. *Euro J Nucl Med* 1998;25:242–6.

101a www.iop.org/search/results?action=search&querytext=urb+%3Ccontains%3E+www.ipem.org.uk

102 Park HM, Park YA, Jhow XH. Detection of thyroid remnant/metastases with stunning – an ongoing dilemma. *Thyroid* 1997;7:277–80.

103 Bal CS, Kumar A, Pant GS. Radioiodine dose for remnant ablation in differentiated thyroid carcinoma: a randomized clinical trial in 509 patients. *J Clin Endocrinol Metab* 2004;89:1666–73.

104 Vini L, Harmer C. Radioiodine treatment for differentiated thyroid cancer. *J Clin Oncol* 2000;12:365–72.

105 Hyer S, Vini L, O'Connell M, Pratt B, Harmer C. Testicular dose and fertility in men following I(131) therapy for thyroid cancer. *Clin Endocrinol (Oxf)* 2002;56:755–8.

106 Thyroid Carcinoma Task Force. *AACE/AAES Medical/surgical guidelines for clinical practice: management of thyroid carcinoma.* Jacksonville, FL: American Association of Clinical Endocrinologists, 2001. www.aace.com/pub/pdf/guidelines/thyroid_carcinoma.pdf

107 Tsang RW, Brierley JD, Simpson WJ *et al.* The effects of surgery, radioiodine and external radiation therapy on the clinical outcome of patients with differentiated thyroid carcinoma. *Cancer* 1998;82:375–88.

108 Brierley J, Tsang R, Panzarella T, Bana N. Prognostic factors and the effect of treatment with radioactive iodine and external beam radiation on patients with differentiated thyroid cancer seen at a single institution over 40 years. *Clin Endocrinol* 2005;63:418–27.

109 Sawka AM, Thephamongkhol K, Brouwers M *et al.* Clinical review 170: A systematic review and metaanalysis of the effectiveness of radioactive iodine remnant ablation for well-differentiated thyroid cancer. *J Clin Endocrinol Metab* 2004;89:3668–76.

110 Hay ID, McConahey WM, Goellner JR. Managing patients with papillary thyroid carcinoma: insights gained from the Mayo Clinic's experience of treating 2,512 consecutive patients during 1940 through 2000. *Trans Am Clin Climatol Assoc* 2002;113:241–60.

111 Rubino C, de Vathaire F, Dottorini ME *et al.* Second primary malignancies in thyroid cancer patients. *Br J Cancer* 2003;89:1638–44.

112 Sandeep TC, Strachan MW, Reynolds RM *et al.* Second primary cancers in thyroid cancer patients: a multinational record linkage study. *J Clin Endocrinol Metab* 2006;91:1819–25.

113 Reiners C, Farahati J. I131 therapy of thyroid cancer patients. *Q J Nucl Med* 1999;43:324–35.

114 Ringel MD, Ladenson PW. Controversies in the follow-up and management of well-differentiated thyroid cancer. *Endocr Relat Cancer* 2004;11:97–116.

115 Bal C, Padhy AK, Jana S, Pant GS, Basu AK. Prospective randomized clinical trial to evaluate the optimal dose of 131 I for remnant ablation in patients with differentiated thyroid carcinoma. *Cancer* 1996;77:2574–80.

116 Sirisalipoch S, Buachum V, Pasawang P, Tepmongkol S. Prospective randomized trial for the evaluation of the efficacy of low vs high dose 131I for post-operative remnant ablation in differentiated thyroid cancer. *World J Nucl Med* 2004;3(Suppl 1):S36.

117 Haq MS, McCready RV, Harmer CL. Treatment of advanced differentiated thyroid carcinoma with high activity radioiodine therapy. *Nucl Med Commun* 2004;25:799–805.

118 Pacini F, Ladenson PW, Schlumberger M *et al.* Radioiodine ablation of thyroid remnants after preparation with recombinant human thyrotropin in differentiated thyroid carcinoma: results of an international, randomized, controlled study. *J Clin Endocrinol Metab* 2006;91:926–32.

119 Fatourechi V, Hay ID, Mullan BP *et al.* Are post therapy radioiodine scans informative and do they influence subsequent therapy of patients with differentiated thyroid cancer? *Thyroid* 2000;10:573–7.

120 Roos DE, Smith JG. Randomized trials on radioactive iodine ablation of thyroid remnants for thyroid carcinoma – a critique. *Int J Radiat Oncol Biol Phys* 1999;44:493–5.

121 Cailleux AF, Baudin E, Travagli JP, Ricard M, Schlumberger M. Is diagnostic iodine-131 scanning useful after total thyroid ablation for differentiated thyroid cancer? *J Clin Endocrinol Metab* 2000;85:175–8.

122 Schlumberger M, Berg G, Cohen O *et al.* Follow-up of low-risk patients with differentiated thyroid carcinoma: a European perspective. *Eur J Endocrinol* 2004;150:105–12.

123 Haugen BR, Pacini F, Reiners C *et al.* A comparison of recombinant human thyrotropin and thyroid hormone withdrawal for the detection of thyroid remnant or cancer. *J Clin Endocrinol Metab* 1999;84:3877–85.

124 Mazzaferri EL, Robbins RJ, Spencer CA *et al.* A consensus report of the role of serum thyroglobulin as a monitoring method for low-risk patients with papillary thyroid carcinoma. *J Clin Endocrinol Metab* 2003;88:1433–41.

125 Administration of Radioactive Substances Advisory Committee. *Notes for guidance on clinical administration of radiopharmaceuticals and use of sealed radioactive sources.* London: HPA, 2006. www.arsac.org.uk/notes_for_guidence/docs/arsac_nfg.pdf

126 Schlumberger M, De Vathaire F, Ceccarelli C *et al.* Exposure to radioactive iodine-131 for scintigraphy or therapy does not preclude pregnancy in thyroid cancer patients. *J Nucl Med* 1996;37:606–12.

127 Ayala C, Navarro E, Rodriguez JR *et al.* Conception after I131 therapy for differentiated thyroid cancer. *Thyroid* 1998;8:1009–11.

128 Dottorini ME, Lomuscio G, Mazzucchelli L, Vignati A, Colombo L. Assessment of female fertility and carcinogenesis after iodine-131 therapy for differentiated thyroid carcinoma. *J Nucl Med* 1995;36:21–7.

129 Bal C, Kumar A, Tripathi M *et al.* High-dose radioiodine treatment for differentiated thyroid carcinoma is not associated with change in female fertility or any genetic risk to the offspring. *Int J Radiat Oncol Biol Phys* 2005;63:449–55.

130 Schroeder PR, Haugen BR, Pacini F *et al.* A comparison of short-term changes in health-related quality of life in thyroid carcinoma patients undergoing diagnostic evaluation with recombinant human thyrotropin compared to thyroid hormone withdrawal. *J Clin Endocrinol Metab* 2006;91:878–84.

131 Schlumberger M, Pacini F. Hazards of medical use of iodine 131. In: *Thyroid tumours.* Paris: Nucleon, 1997:223–35.

132 Simpson WJ, Panzarella T, Carruthers JS, Gospodarowicz MK, Sutcliffe SB. Papillary and follicular thyroid cancer. Impact of treatment in 1578 patients. *Int J Radiat Oncol Biol Phys* 1988;14:1063–75.

133 de Vathaire F, Schlumberger M, Delisle MJ *et al.* Leukaemia and cancers following iodine-131 administration for thyroid cancer. *Br J Cancer* 1997;75:734–9.

134 Dulgeroff AJ, Hershman JM. Medical therapy for differentiated thyroid carcinoma. *Endocr Rev* 1994;15:500–15.

135 Edmonds CJ, Smith T. The long-term hazards of treatment of thyroid cancer with radioiodine. *Br J Radiol* 1986;59:45–51.

136 Brown AP, Greening WP, McCready VR, Shaw HJ, Harmer CL. Radioiodine treatment of metastatic thyroid carcinoma: the Royal Marsden Hospital experience. *Br J Radiol* 1984;57:323–7.

137 Maheshwari YK, Hill CS Jr, Haynie TP 3rd, Hickey RC, Samaan MA. 131I therapy in differentiated thyroid carcinoma: M.D. Anderson Hospital experience. *Cancer* 1981;47:664–71.

138 Rall JE, Alpers JB, Lewallen CG *et al.* Radiation pneumonitis and fibrosis: a complication of radioiodine treatment of pulmonary metastases from cancer of the thyroid. *J Clin Endocrinol Metab* 1957;17:1263–76.

139 Meadows KM, Amdur RJ, Morris CG *et al.* External beam radiotherapy for differentiated thyroid cancer. *Am J Otolaryngol* 2006;27:24–8.

140 Biermann M, Pixberg M, Schuck A *et al.* External beam radiotherapy. In: Biersack H-J, Grünwald F (eds). *Thyroid cancer.* Heidelberg: Springer Verlag, 2005:139–61.

141 Tubiana M, Haddad E, Schlumberger M *et al.* External radiotherapy in thyroid cancers. *Cancer* 1985;55(9 suppl):2062–71.

142 Harmer CL, McCready VR. Thyroid cancer: differentiated carcinoma. *Cancer Treat Rev* 1996;22:161–77.

143 Taylor T, Specker B, Robbins J *et al.* Outcome after treatment of high risk papillary and non-Hurthle-cell follicular thyroid carcinoma. *Ann Intern Med* 1998;129:622–7.

144 Harmer C, Bidmead M, Shepherd S, Sharpe A, Vini L. Radiotherapy planning techniques for thyroid cancer. *Br J Radiol* 1998;71:1069–75.

145 Samaan NA, Schultz PN, Hickey RC *et al.* The results of various modalities of treatment of well differentiated thyroid carcinomas: a retrospective review of 1599 patients. *J Clin Endocrinol Metab* 1992;75:714–20.

146 Hall EJ. The inaugural Frank Ellis Lecture – Iatrogenic cancer: the impact of intensity-modulated radiotherapy. *Clin Oncol (R Coll Radiol)* 2006;18:277–82.

147 Szubin L, Kacker A, Kakani R, Komisar A, Blaugrund S. The management of post-thyroidectomy hypocalcemia. *Ear Nose Throat J* 1996;75:612–4,616.

148 Bentrem DJ, Rademaker A, Angelos P. Evaluation of serum calcium levels in predicting hypoparathyroidism after total/near-total thyroidectomy or parathyroidectomy. *Am Surg* 2001;67:249–51.

149 Chia SH, Weisman RA, Tieu D *et al.* Prospective study of perioperative factors predicting hypocalcemia after thyroid and parathyroid surgery. *Arch Otolaryngol Head Neck Surg* 2006;132:41–5.

150 Thakker RV. Hypocalcemia: pathogenesis, differential diagnosis and management. In: Favus MJ. *Primer on the metabolic bone diseases and disorders of mineral metabolisim*, 5th edn. Washington, DC: American Society of Bone and Mineral Research, 2003:271–4.

151 Biondi B, Filetti S, Schlumberger M. Thyroid-hormone therapy and thyroid cancer: a reassessment. *Nature Clin Pract Endocrinol Metab* 2005;1:32–40.

152 Wang PW, Wang ST, Liu RT *et al.* Levothyroxine suppression of thyroglobulin in patients with differentiated thyroid carcinoma. *J Clin Endocrinol Metab* 1999;84:4549–53.

153 Kamel N, Gullu S, Dagci Ilqin S *et al*. Degree of thyrotropin suppression in differentiated thyroid cancer without recurrence or metastases. *Thyroid* 1999;9:1245–8.

154 Pujol P, Daures JP, Nsakala N *et al*. Degree of thyrotropin suppression as a prognostic determinant in differentiated thyroid cancer. *J Clin Endocrinol Metab* 1996;81:4318–23.

155 Cooper DS, Specker B, Ho M, et al. Thyrotropin suppression and disease progression in patients with differentiated thyroid cancer: results from the National Thyroid Cancer Treatment Cooperative Registry. *Thyroid* 1998;8:737–44.

156 Demers LM, Spencer CA. *Laboratory support for the diagnosis and monitoring of thyroid disease*. Washington, DC: National Academy of Clinical Biochemistry, 2003. www.aacc.org/NR/rdonlyres/F343F1C7-8DFB-4718-A912-030550E087A3/0/3e_thyroid.pdf

157 Spencer CA, Bergoglio LM, Kazarosyan M, Fatemi S, LoPresti JS. Clinical impact of thyroglobulin (Tg) and Tg autoantibody method differences on the management of patients with differentiated thyroid carcinomas. *J Clin Endocrinol Metab* 2005;90:5566–75.

158 Feldt-Rasmussen U, Petersen PH, Date J, Madsen CM. Serum thyroglobulin in patients undergoing subtotal thyroidectomy for toxic and nontoxic goiter. *J Endocrinol Invest* 1982;5:161–4.

159 Izumi M, Kubo I, Taura M *et al*. Kinetic study of immunoreactive human thyroglobulin. *J Clin Endocrinol Metab* 1986;62:410–2.

160 Hocevar M, Auersperg M, Stanovnik L. The dynamics of serum thyroglobulin elimination from the body after thyroid surgery. *Eur J Surg Oncol* 1997;23:208–10.

161 Ozata M, Suzuki S, Miyamoto T *et al*. Serum thyroglobulin in the follow-up of patients with treated differentiated thyroid cancer. *J Clin Endocrinol Metab* 1994;79:98–105.

162 Kloos RT, Mazzaferri EL. A single recombinant human thyrotropin-stimulated serum thyroglobulin measurement predicts differentiated thyroid carcinoma metastases three to five years later. *J Clin Endocrinol Metab* 2005;90:5047–57.

163 Luster M, Lippi F, Jarzab B *et al*. rhTSH-aided radioiodine ablation and treatment of differentiated thyroid carcinoma: a comprehensive review. *Endocr Relat Cancer* 2005;12:49–64.

164 Pacini F, Molinaro E, Castagna MG *et al*. Recombinant human thyrotropin-stimulated serum thyroglobulin combined with neck ultrasonography has the highest sensitivity in monitoring differentiated thyroid carcinoma. *J Clin Endocrinol Metab* 2003;88:3668–73.

165 Kebebew E, Clark OH. Differentiated thyroid cancer 'complete' rational approach. *World J Surg* 2000;24:942–51.

166 Wilson PC, Millar BM, Brierley JD. The management of advanced thyroid cancer. *Clin Oncol* 2004;16:561–8.

167 Van Nostrand D, Atkins F, Yeganeh F *et al*. Dosimetrically determined doses of radioiodine for the treatment of metastatic thyroid carcinoma. *Thyroid* 2002;12:121–34.

168 Sisson JC. Practical dosimetry of I131 in patients with thyroid carcinoma. *Cancer Biother Radiopharm* 2002;17:101–5.

169 McDougall IR. Differentiated thyroid cancer. In: *Management of thyroid cancer and related nodular disease*. Berlin: Springer, 2006:163–82.

170 McDougall IR. Management of thyroglobulin positive/whole-body scan negative: is Tg positive/131I therapy useful? *J Endocrinol Invest* 2001;24:194–8.

171 Ward G, Hickman PE. Phantoms in the assay tube. *J Clin Endocrinol Metab* 2004;89:433.

172 Ma C, Xie J, Kuang A. Is empiric 131I therapy justified for patients with positive Tg and negative 131I whole body scanning results? *J Nucl Med* 2005;46:1164–70.

173 van Tol KM, Jager PL, de Vries EG *et al*. Outcome in patients with differentiated thyroid cancer with negative diagnostic whole-body scanning and detectable stimulated thyroglobulin. *Eur J Endocrinol* 2003;148:589–96.

174 Wang W, Larson SM, Fazzari M *et al*. Prognostic value of [18F]fluorodeoxyglucose positron emission tomographic scanning in patients with thyroid cancer. *J Clin Endocrinl Metab* 2000;85:1107–13.

175 van Tol KM, Jager PL, Piers DA *et al*. Better yield of (18)fluorodeoxyglucose- positron emission tomography in patients with metastatic differentiated thyroid carcinoma during thyrotropin stimulation. *Thyroid* 2002;12:381–7.

176 Wong CO, Dworkin HJ. Role of FDG PET in metastatic thyroid cancer. *J Nucl Med* 1999;40:993–4.

177 Chung JK, So Y, Lee JS *et al*. Value of FDG PET in papillary thyroid carcinoma with negative 131I whole-body scan. *J Nucl Med* 1999;40:986–92.

178 Schluter B, Bohuslaviski KH, Beyer W *et al*. Impact of FDG PET on patients with differentiated thyroid cancer who present with elevated thyroglobulin and negative 131I scan. *J Nucl Med* 2001;42:71–8.

179 Petrich T, Borner AR, Otto D *et al*. Influence of rhTSH on 18-fluorodeoxyglucose uptake by differentiated thyroid carcinoma. *Eur J Nucl Med Mol Imaging* 2002;29:641–7.

180 Stokkel MP, Reigman HI, Verkooijen RB, Smit JW. Indium-111-Octreotide scintigraphy in differentiated thyroid carcinoma metastases that do not respond to treatment with high-dose I-131. *J Cancer Res Clin Oncol* 2003;129:287–94.

181 Teunissen JJ, Kwekkeboom DJ, Kooij PP *et al*. Peptide receptor radionuclide therapy for non radioiodine avid differentiated thyroid cancer. *J Nucl Med* 2005;46:107–14.

182 Mazzaferri EL. Management of differentiated thyroid carcinoma in patients with negative whole-body radioiodine scans and elevated serum thyroglobulin levels. In: Mazzaferri EL, Harmer C, Mallick UK, Kendall-Taylor P (eds). *Practical management of thyroid cancer: a multidisciplinary approach*. London: Springer, 2006:237–54.

183 Schlumberger MJ, Mancusi F, Baudin E, Pacini F. I131 therapy for elevated thyroglobulin levels. *Thyroid* 1997;7:273–5.

184 Carlisle MR, Lu C, McDougall IR. The interpretation of 131I scans in the evaluation of thyroid cancer, with an emphasis on false positive findings. *Nucl Med Commun* 2003;24:715–35.

185 Comisky M. Specialist palliative care for anaplastic thyroid carcinoma. In: Mazzaferri EL, Harmer C, Mallick UK, Kendall-Taylor P (eds). *Practical management of thyroid cancer: a multidisciplinary approach*. London: Springer, 2006:411–9.

186 Shimaoka K, Schoenfeld DA, Dewys WD, Creech RH, De Conti R. A randomized trial of doxorubicin versus doxorubicin plus cisplatin in patients with advanced thyroid cancer. *Cancer* 1985;56:2155–60.

187 Williams SD, Birch R, Einhorn LH. Phase II evaluation of doxorubicin plus cisplatin in advanced thyroid cancer: a Southeastern Cancer Study Group Trial. *Cancer Treat Rep* 1986;70:405–7.

188 Hoskin PJ, Harmer CL. Chemotherapy for thyroid cancer. *Radiother Oncol* 1987;10:187–94.

189 Saller B. Treatment with cytotoxic drugs. In: Biersack H-J, Grünwald F (eds). *Thyroid cancer*. Heidelberg: Springer Verlag, 2005.

190 Moosa M, Mazzaferri EL. Outcome of differentiated thyroid cancer diagnosed in pregnant women. *J Clin Endocrinol Metab* 1997;82:2862–6.

191 Casara D, Rubello D, Saladini G, Piotto G *et al*. Pregnancy after high therapeutic doses of iodine-131 in differentiated thyroid cancer: potential risks and recommendations. *Eur J Nucl Med* 1993;20:192–4.

192 Mandel SJ, Larsen PR, Seely EW, Brent GA. Increased need for thyroxine during pregnancy in women with primary hypothyroidism. *N Engl J Med* 1990;323:91–6.

193 Schlumberger M, De Vathaire F, Travagli JP *et al*. Differentiated thyroid carcinoma in childhood: long term follow-up of 72 patients. *Clin Endocrinol Metab* 1987;65:1088–94.

194 Zimmerman D, Hay ID, Gough IR *et al*. Papillary thyroid carcinoma in children and adults: long-term follow-up of 1039 patients conservatively treated at one institution during three decades. *Surgery* 1988;104:1157–66.

195 Thompson GB, Hay ID. Current strategies for surgical management and adjuvant treatment of childhood papillary thyroid carcinoma. *World J Surg* 2004;28:1187–98.

196 La Quaglia MP, Black T, Holcomb GW *et al*. Differentiated thyroid cancer: clinical characteristics, treatment, and outcome in patients under 21 years of age who present with distant metastases. A report from the Surgical Discipline Committee of the Children's Cancer Group. *J Pediatr Surg* 2000;35:955–9.

197 Jarzab B, Handkiewicz Junak D, Wloch J *et al*. Multivariate analysis of prognostic factors for differentiated thyroid carcinoma in children. *Eur J Nucl Med* 2000;27:833–41.

198 Laundau D, Vini L, Hern RA, Harmer C. Thyroid cancer in children: the Royal Marsden Hospital experience. *Eur J Cancer* 2000;36:214–20.

199 Royal College of Pathologists. *Standards and datasets for reporting cancers: dataset for thyroid cancer histopathology reports*. London: RCPath, 2006. www.rcpath.org/resources/pdf/ThyroidDatasetFeb06.pdf

199a Chen H, Nicol TL, Udelsman R. Follicular lesions of the thyroid. Does frozen section evaluation alter operative management? *Ann Surg* 1995;222:101–6.

200 Udelsman R, Westra WH, Donovan PI, Sohn TA, Cameron JL. Randomized prospective evaluation of frozen-section analysis for follicular neoplasms of the thyroid. *Ann Surg* 2001;233:716–22.

201 Franssila KO, Ackerman LV, Brown CL, Hedinger CE. Follicular carcinoma. *Semin Diagn Pathol* 1985;2:101–22.

202 Hermanek P, Sobin LH (eds). *TNM classification of malignant tumors*, 5th edn. New York: Wiley-Liss, 1992.

203 Royal College of Pathologists. *Standards and datasets for reporting cancers: datasets for histopathology reports on head and neck carcinomas and salivary neoplasms*, 2nd edn. London: RCPath, 2005. www.rcpath.org/resources/pdf/HeadNeckDatasetJun05.pdf

204 Sherman SI. Toward a standard clinicopathologic staging approach for differentiated thyroid carcinoma. *Semin Surg Oncol* 1999;16:12–5.

205 American Joint Committee on Cancer. *AJCC cancer staging manual*, 5th edn. Philadelphia: Lippincott-Raven, 1997.

206 Hay ID, Grant CS, Taylor WF, McConahey WM. Ipsilateral lobectomy versus bilateral lobar resection in papillary thyroid carcinoma: a retrospective analysis of surgical outcome using a novel prognostic scoring system. *Surgery* 1987;102:1088–95.

207 Ogilvie JB, Kebebew E. Indication and timing of thyroid surgery for patients with hereditary medullary thyroid cancer syndromes. *J Natl Compr Canc Netw* 2006;4:139–47.

208 Traugott A, Moley JF. Medullary thyroid cancer: medical management and follow-up. *Curr Treat Options Oncol* 2005;6:339–46.

209 Gagel RF, Cote GJ, Martins Bugalho MJ *et al*. Clinical use of molecular information in the management of multiple endocrine neoplasia type A. *J Intern Med* 1995;238:333–41.

210 Carlson KM, Bracamontes J, Jackson CE *et al*. Parent-of-origin effects in multiple endocrine neoplasia type 2B. *Am J Hum Genet* 1994;55:1076–82.

211 Marsh DJ, McDowall D, Hyland VJ *et al*. The identification of false positive responses to the pentagastrin stimulation test in RET mutation negative members of MEN 2A families. *Clin Endocrinol* 1996;44:213–20.

212 Wells SA, Dilley WG, Farndon JR *et al*. Early diagnosis and treatment of medullary thyroid carcinoma. *Arch Intern Med* 1985;145:1248–52.

213 Raue E, Kraimps JL, Dralle H *et al*. Primary hyperparathyroidism in multiple endocrine neoplasia type 2A. *J Intern Med* 1995;238:369–73.
www.aacc.org/NR/rdonlyres/F343F1C7-8DFB-4718-A912-030550E087A3/0/3e_thyroid.pdf

214 Frilling A, Dralle H, Eng C, Raue F, Broelsch CE. Presymptomatic DNA screening in families with multiple endocrine neoplasia type 2 and familial medullary thyroid carcinoma. *Surgery* 1995;118:1099–104.

215 O'Riordain DS, O'Brien T, Hay ID *et al*. Medullary thyroid carcinoma in multiple endocrine neoplasia type 2A and 2B. *Surgery* 1994;116:1017–23.

216 Pacini F, Romei C, Miccoli P *et al*. Early treatment of hereditary medullary thyroid carcinoma after attribution of multiple endocrine neoplasia type 2 gene carrier status by screening for ret gene mutations. *Surgery* 1995;118:1031–5.

217 Wells SA, Chi DD, Toshima K *et al*. Predictive DNA testing and prophylactic thyroidectomy in patients at risk for multiple endocrine neoplasia type 2. *Ann Surg* 1994;220:237–50.

218 Ukkat J, Gimm O, Brauckhoff M, Bilkenroth U, Dralle H. Single center experience in primary surgery for medullary thyroid carcinoma. *World J Surg* 2004;28:1271–4.

219 Machens A, Holzhausen HJ, Thanh PN, Dralle H. Malignant progression from C-cell hyperplasia to medullary thyroid carcinoma in 167 carriers of RET germline mutations. *Surgery* 2003;134:425–31.

220 van Heurn LW, Schaap C, Sie G *et al*. Predictive DNA testing for multiple endocrine neoplasia 2: a therapeutic challenge of prophylactic thyroidectomy in very young children. *J Pediatr Surg* 1999;34:568–71.

221 de Groot JW, Links TP, Plukker JT, Lips CJ, Hofstra RM. RET as a diagnostic and therapeutic target in sporadic and hereditary endocrine tumors. *Endocr Rev* 2006;27:535–60.

222 Machens A, Ukkat J, Brauckhoff M, Gimm O, Dralle H. Advances in the management of hereditary medullary thyroid cancer. *J Intern Med* 2005;257:50–9.

223 Brandi ML, Gagel RF, Angeli A *et al*. Guidelines for diagnosis and therapy of MEN type 1 and type 2. *J Clin Endocrinol Metab* 2001;86:5658–71.

224 Fugazzola L, Pinchera A, Luchetti F *et al*. Disappearance rate of serum calcitonin after total thyroidectomy for medullary thyroid carcinoma. *Int J Biol Markers* 1994;9:21–4.

225 Dralle H. Lymph node dissection and medullary thyroid carcinoma. *Br J Surg* 2002;89:1073–5.

226 Modigliani E, Franc B, Niccoli-Sire P. Diagnosis and treatment of medullary thyroid cancer. *Baillieres Best Pract Res Clin Endocrinol Metab* 2000;14:631–49.

227 Tung WS, Vesely TM, Moley JF. Laparoscopic detection of hepatic metastases in patients with residual or recurrent medullary thyroid cancer. *Surgery* 1995;118:1024–9.

228 Szavcsur P, Godeny M, Bajzik G *et al*. Angiography-proven liver metastases explain low efficacy of lymph node dissections in medullary thyroid cancer patients. *Eur J Surg Oncol* 2005;31:183–90.

229 Fife KM, Bower M, Harmer C. Medullary thyroid cancer: the role of radiotherapy in local control. *Eur J Surg Oncol* 1996;22:588–91.

230 Hyer SL, Vini L, A'Hern R, Harmer C. Medullary thyroid cancer: multivariate analysis of prognostic factors influencing survival. *Eur J Surg Oncol* 2000;26:686–90.

230 Pinchera A, Elisei R. Medullary thyroid caner: diagnosis and management. In: Mazzaferri EL, Harmer C, Mallick UK, Kendall-Taylor P (eds). *Practical management of thyroid cancer: a multidisciplinary approach*. London: Springer, 2006:255–80.

231 Orlandi F, Caraci P, Berruti A *et al*. Chemotherapy with dacarbazine and 5-fluorouracil in advanced medullary thyroid cancer. *Ann Oncol* 1994;5:763–5.

232 Schlumberger M, Abdelmoumene N, Delisle MJ, Couette JE. Treatment of advanced medullary thyroid cancer with an alternating combination of 5 FU-streptozocin and 5 FU-dacarbazine. The Groupe d'Etude des Tumeurs a Calcitonine (GETC). *Br J Cancer* 1995;71:363–5.

233 Clarke SE, Lazarus CR, Edwards S *et al.* Scintigraphy and treatment of medullary carcinoma of the thyroid with iodine-131 metaiodobenzylguanidine. *J Nucl Med* 1987;28:1820–5.

234 Clarke SE. [131I]metaiodobenzylguanidine therapy in medullary thyroid cancer: Guy's Hospital experience. *J Nucl Biol Med* 1991;35:323–6.

235 Kaltsas G, Rockall A, Papadogias D, Reznek R, Grossman AB. Recent advances in radiological and radionuclide imaging and therapy of neuroendocrine tumours. *Eur J Endocrinol* 2004;151:15–27.

236 Schott M, Seissler J Lettmann M *et al.* Immunotherapy for medullary thyroid carcinoma by dendritic cell vaccination. *J Clin Endocrinol Metab* 2001;86:4965–9.

237 Sala E, Mologni L, Cazzaniga S, Papinutto E, Gambacorti-Passerini C. A rapid method for the purification of wild-type and V804M mutant ret catalytic domain: a tool to study thyroid cancer. *Int J Biol Macromol* 2006;39:60–5.

238 Bolino A, Schuffenecker I, Luo Y *et al.* RET mutations in exons 13 and 14 of FMTC patients. *Oncogene* 1995;10:2415–9.

239 Borrello MG, Smith DP, Pasini B *et al.* RET activation by germline MEN-2A and MEN-2B mutations. *Oncogene* 1995;11:2419–27.

240 Eng C, Clayton D, Schuffenecker I *et al.* The relationship between specific ret protooncogene mutations and disease phenotype in multiple endocrine neoplasia type 2: International RET Mutation Consortium. *JAMA* 1996;276:1575–9.

241 Eng C, Mulligan LM, Smith DP *et al.* Mutation of the RET protooncogene in sporadic medullary thyroid carcinoma. *Genes Chromosomes Cancer* 1995;12:209–12.

242 Lips CJ, Landsvater RM, Hoppener JW *et al.* Clinical screening as compared with DNA analysis in families with multiple endocrine neoplasia type 2A. *N Engl J Med* 1994;331:828–35.

243 Mulligan LM, Eng C, Attie T *et al.* Diverse phenotypes associated with exon 10 mutations of the RET protooncogene. *Hum Mol Genet* 1994;3:2163–7.

244 Mulligan LM, Eng C, Healey CS *et al.* Specific mutations of the RET protooncogene are related to disease phenotype in MEN 2A and FMTC. *Nat Genet* 1994;6:70–4.

245 Mulligan LM, Gardner E, Smith BA *et al.* Genetic events in tumour initiation and progression in multiple endocrine neoplasia type 2. *Genes Chromosomes Cancer* 1993;6:166–77.

246 Mulligan LM, Kwok JB, Healey CS *et al.* Germline mutations of the RET proto-oncogene in multiple endocrine neoplasia type 2A. *Nature* 1993;363:458–60.

247 Mulligan LM, Marsh DJ, Robinson BG *et al.* Genotype-phenotype correlation in MEN 2; report of the international RET mutations consortium. *J Intern Med* 1995;238:343–6.

248 Farndon JR, Leight GS, Dilley WG *et al.* Familial medullary thyroid carcinoma without associated endocrinopathies: a distinct clinical entity. *Br J Surg* 1986;73:278–81.

249 Russell CF, Van Heerden JA, Sizemore GW *et al.* The surgical management of medullary thyroid carcinoma. *Ann Surg* 1983;197:42–8.

250 O'Riordain DS, O'Brien T, Crotty TB *et al.* Multiple endocrine neoplasia type 2B: more than an endocrine disorder. *Surgery* 1995;118:936–42.

251 Samaan NA, Draznin MB, Halpin RE *et al.* Multiple endocrine syndrome type IIB in early childhood. *Cancer* 1991;68:1832–4.

252 Carlson KM, Dou S, Chi D *et al.* Single missense mutation in the tyrosine kinase catalytic domain of the RET protooncogene is associated with multiple endocrine neoplasia type 2B. *Proc Natl Acad Sci USA* 1994;91:1579–83.

253 Toogood AA, Eng C, Smith DP *et al.* No mutation at codon 918 of the RET gene in a family with multiple endocrine neoplasia type 2B. *Clin Endocrinol* 1995;43:759–62.

254 International Atomic Energy Agency. *International criteria in a nuclear or nuclear radiation emergency. Safety Series 109.* Vienna: IAEA, 1991.

255 International Commission on Radiological Protection. *ICRP publication 63. Principles for intervention for protection of the public in a radiological emergency.* Oxford: Pergamon Press, 1991.

256 Spencer CA. Challenges of serum thyroglobulin (Tg) measurement in the presence of Tg autoantibodies. *J Clin Endocrinol Metab* 2004;89:3702–4.

257 Stockigt JR. Ambiguous thyroglobulin assay results in the follow-up of differentiated thyroid carcinoma. *J Clin Endocrinol Metab* 2005;90:5904–5.

258 Weightman DR, Mallick UK, Fenwick JD, Perros P. Discordant serum thyroglobulin results generated by two classes of assay in patients with thyroid carcinoma: correlation with clinical outcome after 3 years of follow-up. *Cancer* 2003;98:41–7.

Appendix 5 Patient information

Patient representatives have been fully involved in each stage of development of the guidelines and the patient information literature.

1 Patient support groups

Cancerbackup
3 Bath Place
Rivington Street
London
EC2A 3JR
www.cancerbackup.org.uk
Tel: 020 7696 9003
Freephone: 0808 800 1234

Butterfly North East
PO Box 205
Rowlands Gill
Tyne & Wear
NE39 2WX
butterflynortheast@btopenworld.com
Tel: 01207 545469

Thyroid Cancer Support UK
www.thyroidcancersupportuk.org/

British Thyroid Foundation
PO Box 97
Clifford
Wetherby
West Yorkshire
LS23 6XD
www.btf-thyroid.org
Tel: 01423 709707/709448

Association for Multiple Endocrine Neoplasia Disorders – AMEND (MEN2/FMTC)
31 Pennington Place
Southborough
Kent
TN4 0AQ
email: jo.grey@amend.org.uk

2 Websites with useful information for patients

British Thyroid Foundation
www.btf-thyroid.org

AMEND (information re MEN syndromes)
www.amend.org.uk

Cancerbackup
www.cancerbackup.org.uk

Butterfly North East
www.butterfly.org.uk

Thyroid Foundation of America
www.tsh.org/

Cancernet
www.thyroid-cancer.net/

Medline (search the medical literature)
www.medlineplus.gov/

Medline (information for patients)
www.nlm.nih.gov/medlineplus/ency/article/001213.htm

Thyroid Cancer Survivors' Association
www.thyca.org/

The thyroid gland and thyroid cancer

Your tests and treatment

The thyroid gland

What is the thyroid gland?

The thyroid gland is an endocrine gland and makes hormones which are released into the bloodstream. These hormones affect cells and tissues in other parts of the body and help them to function normally.

Where is the thyroid gland?

The thyroid gland is at the base of the throat. It is made up of two lobes (each about half the size of a plum). The two lobes lie on either side of your windpipe, with the gland as a whole lying just below your Adam's apple. The thyroid gland and windpipe (with a cross-section of it above the thyroid lobes) are shown below.

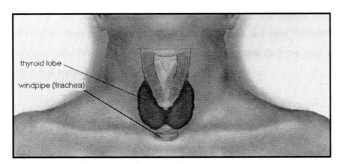

thyroid lobe

windpipe (trachea)

What does the thyroid gland do?

The thyroid gland produces three hormones that are released into the bloodstream:

- Thyroxine, often called T4.
- Triiodothyronine, often called T3. In the body, T4 is converted into T3 and this is what influences the way cells and tissues work.
- Calcitonin. This is involved in controlling calcium levels in the blood. With medullary thyroid cancer (MTC), too much calcitonin is produced.

Thyroxine and T3 can both be replaced by medication, and the body can function perfectly well with little or no calcitonin.

What do the thyroid hormones do?

Thyroid hormones (T3 and T4) help to control the speed of body processes – your metabolic rate. If too much of the thyroid hormones is released, your body works faster than normal and you have 'hyperthyroidism'. This would make you feel overactive and anxious, hungrier than usual, and you would lose weight. However, if too little of the thyroid hormones is produced, your body works slower than normal and you have 'hypothyroidism'. In that case, you would feel tired and sluggish, and put on weight easily.

How is the thyroid gland controlled?

Most glands work together with other glands, and the thyroid gland works with the pituitary gland. The thyroid is controlled by the pituitary, which lies underneath your brain in your skull and senses the levels of thyroid hormones in your bloodstream. If the levels drop below normal, the pituitary reacts by releasing a hormone called the 'thyroid-stimulating hormone' or TSH. TSH stimulates the thyroid gland to produce more T3 and T4. If the thyroid hormone levels rise above normal levels, the pituitary senses this and stops releasing TSH and so the thyroid gland will produce less T3 and T4.

How is thyroid activity measured?

Your doctor will be able to get a good assessment of your thyroid gland activity by taking a history of your symptoms and by a physical examination. However, to gain an exact level of the thyroid hormones, it is necessary to take a small sample of blood, which when analysed in the laboratory will show how much T4 and T3 are being produced, and how active your pituitary is, by measuring the level of TSH. These tests are sometimes called thyroid function tests or TFTs.

What are the parathyroid glands and how do they affect calcium levels?

Next to the thyroid gland is another set of glands called the parathyroid glands. There are normally four parathyroids, although this can sometimes vary. The parathyroids produce parathyroid hormone (PTH) and this controls the amount of calcium in the blood. Normal calcium levels in the blood are essential for healthy bones, blood clotting, cardiac rhythm and function of the cells, as well as for general well-being. Too much calcium can make you feel sick and drowsy; too little can cause problems with the nerves such as pins and needles, and make your muscles twitch and jerk.

Thyroid cancer

Most cancers of the thyroid gland are very slow growing and it may be many years before the symptoms become obvious.

Are all thyroid cancers the same?

No, there are different types:

- **Papillary carcinoma** – this is the most common thyroid cancer. It is more common in younger people, particularly women.
- **Follicular carcinoma** – this is less common, and tends to occur in slightly older people than those with papillary cancer.
- **Medullary carcinoma** – this is a rare cancer, which is sometimes hereditary (ie it is passed down through a family from one generation to the next).

Most thyroid cancers are very treatable and curable, but it is possible that they will recur, especially in the very young and very old. This can occur at any stage, but recurrences **can** be treated successfully, so lifelong follow-up is most important.

What is the cause of thyroid cancer?

The cause of thyroid cancer is unknown, but exposure to radiation is known to increase the risk of getting thyroid cancer. For example, after the Chernobyl accident, many more children in the area got thyroid cancer. Similarly, it has been found in people who had external radiotherapy to the neck 10 or 20 years earlier. Research into the causes of thyroid cancer is ongoing. Very occasionally papillary cancer is hereditary, and medullary cancer is quite often hereditary.

What are the symptoms of thyroid cancer?

- A painless lump in the neck which gradually increases in size.
- Difficulty in swallowing (dysphagia) – because of pressure of the enlarged thyroid gland on the oesophagus (gullet).
- Difficulty in breathing (dyspnoea) – because of pressure of the enlarged thyroid gland on the trachea (windpipe).
- Hoarseness of the voice.
- Symptoms of hyperthyroidism (overactive thyroid) and hypothyroidism (underactive thyroid) are rare, as cancer cells do not generally affect hormone production from the thyroid.

Often there are no symptoms and it is found 'by chance'.

What tests will I need?

If you have one of the above symptoms, you will need further tests to check the diagnosis. Your GP will do a blood test to see if your thyroid hormone levels are within normal limits. This test on its own will not show whether you have cancer, but it will help your GP decide which specialist you need to see next. Many of the special tests that will help doctors make a diagnosis will be done in a specialist hospital clinic.

Fine needle aspiration. This is done in an outpatient hospital clinic. A very small needle is inserted into any swelling you may have in your neck and a sample of cells is taken out. These cells are then analysed under a microscope. This is one of the main tests that will help clarify your diagnosis.

Blood test. Some additional blood tests may be done to re-check the function of your thyroid and your levels of thyroid antibodies.

Ultrasound scan. In this test, a picture of the thyroid gland is obtained by using sound waves and it will show any solid lumps or cysts. Again, this on its own cannot diagnose cancer but it can help with the overall diagnosis and in planning treatment.

Radioisotope scan. This type of scan is occasionally helpful in assessing thyroid lumps. A tiny dose of radioactive iodine is given as a capsule (or alternatively another radioactive substance called 'technetium' is given as an injection); then after a short time a gamma camera is placed over the neck.

The camera measures the amount of radioactive substance taken up by the thyroid gland. Cancer cells do not absorb radioactive substances as well as normal thyroid cells, so a small cancer may show on the scan as a 'cold' nodule. However it is not a very good diagnostic test and many so-called 'cold' nodules are benign, not cancerous.

What treatment will I be offered?

You may be offered surgery (thyroidectomy)

Surgery is usually the first line of treatment for thyroid cancer. Usually the whole thyroid gland (total thyroidectomy) will need to be removed, though sometimes only one lobe has to be removed; it depends on various factors such as your age, the size of the lump and results of the tests mentioned above. The parathyroid glands may or may not be removed. After a thyroidectomy, you will need to take thyroxine tablets as prescribed for the rest of your life; regular blood tests will be needed to check that your thyroid hormone levels are within normal limits, and that the TSH level is suppressed. Eventually you should only need a blood test once or twice a year.

Following surgery you will need to have your hormone levels monitored

After your thyroid surgery, your GP will need to monitor your thyroid medication and get blood tests to check your hormone levels. When you are at home after your surgery, please contact your GP or treatment centre if:

▪ you feel extremely tired
▪ you have feelings of pins and needles in your hands, feet or face
▪ you have palpitations
▪ you feel shaky
▪ you become very overactive, or
▪ you generally feel very unwell.

This may mean you need to have your thyroxine or calcium levels checked and your medication dose increased or decreased, as the case may be. Once your body has settled you will be able to lead a normal life but you will need to continue to take the thyroxine tablets for the rest of your life and to have your thyroid levels checked regularly. It will be particularly important to have your thyroid

hormones (TSH) checked if you become pregnant, as you may need to increase your dose of thyroxine (levothyroxine).

You will probably also need to have radioactive iodine treatment

Most people need to have radioactive iodine treatment after surgery to destroy any remaining thyroid or cancer cells. Your doctor will tell you if this is the case. Radioactive iodine treatment is painless – it means taking either one or two capsule-type tablets, or as a liquid, in a single dose. You should not feel sick or lose any hair or have any other side effects with the usual dose required. It is a low dose of radiation but, for the safety of others, for the first 2–4 days a person needs to come into hospital and reduce their social contact. If you need this treatment you will be informed by your specialist consultant and given an information booklet like this one before you start treatment.

Most thyroid cancers are very treatable and curable

Please contact your specialist treatment centre staff or your GP if you have any questions or concerns after reading this information booklet. Together we can help you through your investigations, treatment and recovery.

Useful contacts

The British Thyroid Foundation
PO Box 97, Clifford, Wetherby, West Yorkshire LS23 6XD
Tel: 01423 709707/01423 709448
www.btf-thyroid.org

Butterfly Northeast
PO Box 205, Rowlands Gill, Tyne & Wear NE39 2WX
Tel: 01207 545469
www.butterfly.org.uk

Thyroid Cancer Support UK
www.thyroidcancersupportuk.org/

Association for Multiple Endocrine Neoplasia Disorders AMEND (MEN2/FMTC)
31 Pennington Place, Southborough, Kent TN4 0AQ
www.amend.org.uk
email: jo.grey@amend.org.uk

Cancerbackup
3 Bath Place, Rivington Street, London EC2A 3JR
Tel: 0808 800 1234
www.cancerbackup.org.uk

Macmillan Cancer Support
89 Albert Embankment, London SE1 7UQ
Freephone 0808 808 2020
www.macmillan.org.uk/home.aspx

Cancerlink
Freephone Information Helpline: 0800 132905
www.personal.u-net.com/~njh/cancer.html

CancerHelp UK
www.cancerhelp.org.uk/

Thyroid Cancer Survivors' Association
www.thyca.org/

Other useful sites can be found in the **British Thyroid Association links page:**
www.btf-thyroid.org/

Patient Information Leaflet 2
Thyroid surgery for cancer
Your thyroidectomy

What is a thyroidectomy?

A thyroidectomy is the removal of the whole thyroid gland ('total thyroidectomy') or part of it ('hemithyroidectomy' or 'lobectomy'). You may need to have this done because you have a swelling or enlarged gland or for thyroid cancer treatment. Your specialist will explain to you whether a part or all of your thyroid needs to be removed, so that you can give fully informed consent. If you do not understand any of the information you are given, please ask, as it is very important for you to make the right decision.

Is it a safe operation and what are the side effects?

Thyroid surgery is safe. Before the operation you will be examined and have some additional tests in order to make sure you are fit enough to have a general anaesthetic. Even if you have other medical conditions such as heart or chest trouble, it is usually safe to have the operation.

- The total removal of the thyroid gland means that you will need to take replacement hormone tablets called thyroxine every day for the rest of your life, otherwise you will experience symptoms of hypothyroidism (underactive thyroid). Thyroxine tablets are the size of a sugar sweetener and safe to take. With monitoring by your specialist centre and/or your GP you should be able to lead an active and normal life.

- Thyroxine tablets are also given to suppress the level of thyroid-stimulating hormone (TSH). This is an important part of the treatment for thyroid cancer so most patients will be given thyroxine even if they have had only part of the thyroid removed. You will be advised on this before you go home from hospital.

- You will need regular blood tests to measure the levels of hormones in your blood, and your medication will be adjusted accordingly. You will be given appointments for this.

- Thyroidectomy does not affect your ability to have children, but if you are thinking of starting a family do ask your specialist for advice and information first.

Will it affect my voice?

The thyroid gland lies close to the voice box (larynx) and the nerves to the voice box. After your surgery you may find that your voice sounds hoarse and weak and your singing voice may be slightly altered, but this generally recovers quite quickly. In a very small number of cases voice change can be permanent.

Will my calcium levels be affected following thyroid surgery?

The parathyroid glands control the levels of calcium in the blood and are found close to the thyroid. Sometimes these glands are affected during surgery; if that is the case you may experience tingling sensations in your hands, fingers, in your lips or around your nose. Sometimes people may feel quite unwell. Please report this to the staff looking after you or, if you are at home, to your GP. Blood tests will be taken to monitor the levels of calcium in your blood following surgery. If the level of calcium is falling this can easily be treated by giving you calcium supplements, which may be given through a drip and/or by tablets. You may only need to take these tablets temporarily as the parathyroids usually get back to normal after removal of the thyroid. The medical and nursing staff will advise you about this.

Will I have neck stiffness, restricted shoulder movement or pain?

You will feel some discomfort and stiffness around your neck but you will be given some medication to help ease any pain and discomfort. Pain relief may be given in different ways, such as injections, liquid medicine or tablets. Most patients say the discomfort is not as bad as they expected and after the first day they are up and walking around. Two days after your surgery you will be given some gentle neck exercises to do; this may be given in an information sheet but please do ask staff if you are unsure what to do. After a few weeks your neck and shoulder movements should be back to normal.

Will I have a scar?

Whether all or part of your thyroid has been removed, you will have a scar, but once this is healed it is usually not very noticeable. The scar runs in the same direction as the natural lines of the skin on your neck.

When will the operation be done?

If you have been to an outpatient clinic you may have been given a date for your operation at that time. Otherwise you may receive a date through the post or by phone from your consultant's secretary.

What happens in a pre-admission assessment clinic?

Some hospitals (not all) run a pre-admission assessment clinic, and you may be invited to go there one or two weeks before your operation. This enables both the doctors and the nurses to assess your health needs and carry out routine tests which may be needed before surgery, such as blood tests, a heart tracing (ECG) and a chest X-ray.

The pre-admission assessment gives you the opportunity to meet the ward staff and to see where you will be admitted on the day of your operation. It is also a time when you can ask questions and discuss any concerns you may have about your operation and coming into hospital.

Time is allocated for each individual and you should expect to be there no longer than two hours. However, in unusual circumstances a delay may be unavoidable.

Some patients may have their tests carried out the day before surgery and in that case would not be asked to attend a pre-admission assessment.

What about smoking?

All hospitals operate a 'No Smoking' policy and smoking is not allowed on the ward. If you do smoke, it is in your own health interests to stop smoking at least 24 hours before your anaesthetic.

Please contact your GP's surgery for advice on stopping smoking.

What shall I bring into hospital?

Please bring nightwear, day wear, dressing gown, towels, toiletries, slippers, books/magazines and a pen. It will be helpful to arrange for a relative or friend to wash your nightwear etc and bring in fresh supplies. Hospital nightwear is available if required.

You must bring with you any medication you are currently taking, including inhalers.

Please do not bring any valuables with you, such as jewellery, large sums of money or bank cards. The hospital cannot take responsibility for your valuables. On your admission you will be asked to sign a disclaimer form which gives you the responsibility for any valuables you bring with you. Valuables may be taken for temporary safe keeping by the ward staff while you have your operation and you will be given a receipt.

Will there be a bed ready when I arrive?

Because the hospital runs an emergency service, it is not always possible to predict how many beds will be available. Also, operations are carried out every day and patients are discharged home every day. It is therefore difficult to predict early in the morning how many beds will be available.

You may be asked to take a seat in the waiting room until your bed is ready. You may be waiting for another person who has already had an operation to be discharged. The operation lists are planned and it is necessary to operate in a certain order due to many circumstances. That is why beds are allocated in order of operating lists and not in order of arrival. Please feel free to ask any member of staff for help and advice at any time. Hospital staff will do their best to accommodate you and to keep you waiting for as little time as possible.

What instructions or help will I have to get ready for surgery?

When you have been taken to your bed, the nurse will welcome you and check your details. You will need to wear a special theatre gown for your operation. This will be given to you by the nurse who will show you how to wear it and help you if you want.

Please only wear cotton pants/underpants under your gown. All other underwear must be removed to ensure your safety while equipment is used in the operating theatre.

You will also be given a pair of white elastic stockings to wear during and after the operation which will prevent blood clots from forming in your legs. They feel quite tight and you may need help in putting them on.

What preparation will I need for the operation?

Your operation will be carried out under a general anaesthetic which means that you will be fully unconscious for the whole operation. Removing all or part of the thyroid involves delicate surgery which means that the operation can take about two hours.

To prevent vomiting and other complications during your operation you will be asked not to eat or drink anything for at least six hours before your operation. You will be told what time to start this period without eating food or drink when you attend the pre-admission assessment or by letter from the consultant's secretary.

You should expect to be in hospital for about four days, or longer if any complications arise.

If you would like to meet another patient who has had a thyroidectomy this can sometimes be arranged.

What will happen when I go to theatre?

Just before going to theatre a nurse will complete a checklist. You will then be taken on your bed to the operating theatre, usually by a theatre technician and a nurse. The nurse will stay with you in the anaesthetic room.

Dentures, glasses and hearing aids can be removed in the anaesthetic room and taken back to the ward by the nurse, or you may like to put them in your locker before your operation.

The anaesthetist will insert a small needle into the back of your hand and give you your anaesthetic through that. The nurse will stay with you until you are fully under the anaesthetic and fully asleep. You will not wake up until the operation is over. You will be taken, on your bed, to the recovery area where a nurse will look after you until you are awake. You will then be taken back to the ward, on your bed, by a theatre technician and a nurse.

What will happen when I get back on the ward following surgery?

Back on the ward you will be made comfortable. You will be sitting fairly upright in your bed supported by several pillows as this will help to reduce any neck swelling. Your nurse call bell will be situated close to you so that you can call a nurse at any time.

You will have your blood pressure, pulse and oxygen levels checked frequently. A machine will do this automatically – a blood pressure cuff is wrapped around your upper arm and a probe is clipped to one of your fingers.

There will be a fluid drip going into a vein, probably in the back of your hand; this will be removed as soon as you are drinking normally (usually within 24 hours). You will be able to sip drinks quite soon after your operation as long as you are not feeling sick, and you can eat as soon as you feel able.

What will I look like after thyroid surgery and what will I be able to do?

You will have a scar on the front part of your neck which will feel a little tight and swollen initially after the operation. It may feel a bit sensitive but should not cause any distress.

You may have one or two wound drains from your wound to collect wound fluid which naturally occurs after your surgery. The drains are small plastic tubes which are inserted into the neck at the end of your operation. The long length of tubing outside the neck is attached to a plastic bottle that collects the fluid. Wound drains help to speed up healing and reduce infection. The drains are not painful and you can carry them around with you. They will be removed by a nurse usually a day or two after your operation when there is very little fluid coming through.

You will feel some discomfort and stiffness around your neck but you will be given some medication to help ease any pain and discomfort. Pain relief may be given in different ways such as injections, liquid medicine or tablets. Most patients say it was not as bad as they expected and after the first day they are up and walking around.

For your own safety it is important that you do not get out of bed on your own immediately after your operation as you may be drowsy and weak. At first when you need to use the toilet a member of staff will need to help you with a commode or bedpan. You will soon be able to walk to the bathroom yourself.

You will have a nurse call bell within easy reach so that you can get help from the ward staff as needed.

After your operation you may not feel very sociable so it is wise to restrict visitors.

Will it affect my eating and drinking?

For a short period after your operation you may find it painful to swallow and you may need a softer diet. You may find that nutritious drinks are helpful in providing a balanced diet which is important to assist healing.

Will I have a sore neck?

You will probably find that your neck is quite sore and you will be given painkillers to take home to relieve the discomfort. Please take your painkillers as described on the packet and take care not to exceed the recommended number of tablets. The painkillers should also ease the discomfort caused by swallowing. Your neck may appear swollen and hard to touch, with some numbness, which will gradually ease as healing takes place.

What should I do to reduce any risk of wound infection?

Keep your neck wound clean and dry. Initially the nursing staff will check your wound daily and clean it as necessary. A few days after surgery when you are feeling better you may have a shower or bath but take care to ask the nursing staff's advice first and gently pat the wound dry with a clean towel. Exposure to the air will assist wound healing.

If your neck becomes increasingly painful, red or swollen or you notice any discharge then please seek medical advice from ward staff or your GP. To reduce the risk of infection it is wise to avoid crowded places and take extra care of yourself. Use only clean towels on your wound area for the first few weeks.

What care do I need to take regarding my neck wound?

Take care not to knock your wound and remember to keep it dry if it becomes wet after bathing or showering by patting it dry with a clean towel. Once the scar has begun to heal, you can rub a small amount of unscented moisturising cream on the scar so it is less dry as it heals. Calendula, aloe vera or E45 cream (available from health shops) is effective. The pressure of rubbing the cream in will also help to soften the scar.

What rest do I need?

You will need to take it easy while your neck wound is healing. This means avoiding strenuous activity and heavy lifting for a couple of weeks. Your neck will gradually feel less stiff and you will soon be able to enjoy your normal activities.

What about my medication and tablets?

Please continue to take the medication you have been prescribed and ensure that you have a good supply. If you are unsure about any of the tablets you need to take, please check this with a nurse before you go home. Repeat prescriptions can be obtained from your GP. When you go for your appointments at the hospital to check your blood levels after your surgery, your medication may need to be altered so please check with the medical staff.

When should I return to work?

You will probably need to take about three weeks off work (or sometimes longer), depending on your occupation and the nature of your work. The hospital can issue you with a note for two weeks and then you should see your GP if more time is needed.

Will I need to be checked in an outpatient department following discharge home?

Following your discharge you will need to be reviewed in the outpatient clinic to check how your wound is settling down, your hormone levels and how you are feeling. You will usually receive the date and time for this appointment through the post or it may be given to you by the ward staff before you go home. Please contact the ward or the consultant's secretary at the hospital if you do not receive an appointment shortly after discharge. Depending on the problem with your thyroid and the results from the thyroid tissue that has been removed, you may be offered further treatment. This will be discussed with you by your specialist consultant at your clinic appointment. If you would like any further information, please do not hesitate to ask the nursing staff.

Will I be able to cope?

When most people are first told they need to have a thyroidectomy, they say they feel all sorts of mixed emotions; some might feel numb, and others say they knew all the time that they would need surgery. We are all individuals and cope in different ways so we need different lengths of time to adjust to the changes we face.

> **You do not have to face your treatment on your own.**
> **Support and help is available from the staff.**
> **Together we can help you through your investigations, treatment and recovery.**

Useful contacts

The British Thyroid Foundation
PO Box 97, Clifford, Wetherby, West Yorkshire LS23 6XD
Tel: 01423 709707/01423 709448
www.btf-thyroid.org

Butterfly Northeast
PO Box 205, Rowlands Gill, Tyne & Wear NE39 2WX
Tel: 01207 545469
www.butterfly.org.uk

Thyroid Cancer Support UK
www.thyroidcancersupportuk.org

Association for Multiple Endocrine Neoplasia Disorders AMEND (MEN2/FMTC)
31 Pennington Place, Southborough, Kent TN4 0AQ
www.amend.org.uk
email: jo.grey@amend.org.uk

Cancerbackup
Bath Place, Rivington Street, London EC2A 3JR
Tel: 0808 800 1234
www.cancerbackup.org.uk

Macmillan Cancer Support
89 Albert Embankment, London SE1 7UQ
Freephone: 0808 808 2020
www.macmillan.org.uk/home.aspx

Cancerlink
Freephone Information Helpline: 0800 132905
www.personal.u-net.com/~njh/cancer.html

CancerHelp UK
www.cancerhelp.org.uk

Thyroid Cancer Survivors' Association
www.thyca.org

Other useful sites can be found in the **British Thyroid Association links page:**
www.btf-thyroid.org

Patient Information Leaflet 3
Radioactive iodine ablation and therapy
Things you need to know

Radioactive iodine 'ablation' is treatment with radioactive iodine, which is used to kill off any remaining thyroid tissue in the neck after a thyroid operation. Radioactive iodine 'therapy' refers to treatment with radioactive iodine which is used to kill off thyroid cancer cells in the neck or elsewhere in the body. Radioactive iodine therapy is given only if the tests show that there are still cancer cells in the body.

Most of what follows applies to both 'ablation' and 'therapy' and will be referred to as 'radioactive iodine treatment'.

This form of treatment (ablation or therapy) consists of swallowing radioactive iodine either as a capsule or a liquid. The radioactive iodine is taken up by the thyroid gland. The small dose of radiation is then concentrated in the thyroid cells and destroys them. To receive radioactive iodine ablation or treatment, you will need to be admitted into hospital and stay in a special room (called the iodine suite) so that the radioactivity that your body will be excreting can be safely contained.

Is radioactive iodine treatment (ablation or therapy) safe?

Radioactive iodine has been used to treat thyroid cancer for over 50 years. The greatest danger from radioactive iodine is to the thyroid gland but, as your thyroid has been removed, it is not at risk; the treatment is meant to destroy any thyroid cells that may have escaped surgical removal. Radioactive iodine treatment has been linked with an increased risk of developing other cancers, but this risk is small and has to be balanced against the benefits in treating the thyroid cancer. Your treatment team will discuss these issues with you in detail before the treatment.

The precautions described below are intended to protect other people, particularly pregnant women and young children. It makes sense to reduce everyone's exposure to radioactivity, as any one of us may need this form of treatment in the future.

Are there any side effects from radioactive iodine treatment?

Most patients do not have side effects from radioactive iodine treatment. Some patients may experience a feeling of tightness or swelling in the throat and/or feel flushed, which usually lasts for no more than 24 hours. If this goes on longer, please inform the nursing staff, as an anti-inflammatory drug can be given to relieve this problem. Sometimes having radioactive iodine can result in a temporary taste disturbance, which can last for a few weeks. Drinking plenty of fluids after the treatment helps to wash out the radioactivity and reduce this problem. Please do talk through any of your questions with the specialist consultant or a member of the treatment team.

What if I am pregnant or breastfeeding?

It is very important that you **do not have radioactive iodine treatment if you are pregnant or think there is a good chance that you may be.** Please let your treatment team know if you are unsure before you have any treatment. It is important not to become pregnant when having investigations for thyroid cancer. You should use a reliable contraceptive during investigations, treatment and for at least 6 months after radioactive iodine treatment. In the long term, your fertility will not be affected even after repeated doses of radioactive iodine.

If you are breastfeeding, you should stop this at least four weeks and preferably eight weeks before you have the radioactive iodine treatment and you should not start again afterwards.

(Male patients) Will it affect my ability to have children?

Male patients are advised not to try for children (get their partners pregnant) for four months after radioactive iodine treatment and until they are sure they will not need any more radioactive iodine treatment. In the long term your fertility should not be affected but there may be a small risk if repeated radioactive iodine therapy is needed. Please discuss this with your specialist consultant or a member of the treatment team before trying for a family after this treatment: specialist advice and help is available.

Before having radioactive iodine treatment, what medication/tablets should I take?

If you are taking **T3 (triiodothyronine) tablets**, most specialist centres recommend that these should be stopped for **two weeks** before your radioactive iodine treatment.

If you are on **levothyroxine tablets**, most specialist centres will advise you to stop taking them for **four weeks** before the radioactive iodine treatment. In this four-week period your specialist may first change you to T3 tablets for 2 weeks, and then stop your tablets altogether for the last two weeks before your treatment. You may feel weak and tired when you are not taking your tablets. This is normal and will disappear once you start taking them again, usually a few days after you have had your radioactive iodine.

It is important that you follow the instructions about stopping your thyroxine medication given to you by your specialist centre staff as it may vary in different centres. If you are unsure about your thyroxine medication, please contact your specialist centre **one month before your planned date for radioactive iodine treatment.**

Should I keep taking my other medication/tablets?

If you are taking any other tablets you should carry on doing so and bring a supply with you on admission and show them to the doctor and nurse team. If you are taking any vitamin or mineral supplements or cod liver oil, you should stop taking them around three weeks before your therapy to help reduce your iodine levels.

Before my radioactive iodine therapy what should I eat?

A diet which is rich in iodine can **reduce** the effectiveness of the treatment. Therefore, two weeks before coming in to hospital we recommend the following:

- **Do eat** fresh meat, vegetables, fresh fruit, pasta and rice. These are low in iodine.

- **Do not eat** glacé and maraschino cherries which contain the colouring material E127. Food coloured by spices is allowed.

- **Do not take** cough medicine, iodised table salt or sea salt, as these contain iodine. Ordinary table salt is allowed.

- **Try to cut down on** dairy produce such as eggs, cheese, milk and milk products as they all contain some iodine.

- **Avoid** fish, kelp and all seafood.

- **Avoid** vitamin supplements which contain iodine.

Do I have to come into hospital for radioactive iodine treatment?

Yes, you will probably need to stay in hospital for 3–6 days. How soon you go home depends on how quickly the radioactivity leaves your body.

What happens on admission?

On the ward you will be greeted and your details will be registered. You will then be given a hospital name band to wear, with your hospital registration number and a few details on it. One of the nursing staff will take your blood pressure, pulse and temperature as a routine procedure. You will be given an explanation of the treatment and details about the room where you will be staying. You will also have the opportunity to ask any questions that you might have.

Your doctor will then come to examine you and check that you have stopped taking your thyroid tablets before the treatment as this interferes with the absorption of the radioactive iodine. You will have been sent information about this with your appointment letter.

You will be asked to sign a form giving consent for the treatment.

Who gives the capsule?

The nuclear medicine (or medical physics) department within the hospital is responsible for dealing with the radioactive iodine treatment. One of their staff will come to the ward to give you the capsule (which is about the size of an antibiotic capsule) or the liquid (which is colourless and tasteless.

What happens next?

For the first two hours after taking the capsule you should not eat or drink anything to allow time for the iodine to be absorbed. After this time you should eat as normal and drink as much as possible so that you pass urine frequently. This will flush the excess radioactive iodine out of your system.

Are there any restrictions?

As the treatment you have received is radioactive, no young children or pregnant women will be allowed to visit. Others may visit for a short time. Because you are *radioactive*, staff will spend only short periods of time in your room. When they bring in your meals and drinks they may stand behind a lead screen and you should try to stay on the opposite side of the room. Do not expect them to stay and chat for long periods of time but do not hesitate to contact them if you need anything.

What happens at meal times?

The nursing staff will bring you meals in your room. These meals may be served on paper plates and you may need to use plastic cutlery. When you have finished your meal these should be thrown away in a bin provided. If there is any unwanted food this needs to be sealed in a plastic bag and put in the bin. Alternatively, if ordinary plates and cutlery are used, these will have to be washed up either in your room or in a special kitchen. A waste disposal unit may be available to dispose of any unwanted food. Each day you will receive a menu to fill in for the next day. Drinks are provided in the morning, mid-morning, lunch time, tea time and night-time. If you do not receive your meal for whatever reason please ring the nurses' station, and they will provide you with one. We will try our best to ensure that this does not happen.

What about washing and hygiene?

As you should be drinking a lot, you should also be using the toilet frequently. All your bodily fluids are radioactive so you must flush the toilet after use. If you spill or splash urine please contact the nursing staff.

Your sweat is also radioactive, so we advise you take a bath or shower daily.

What can I can bring in with me to help me relax or pass the time?

You can bring DVDs, CDs, laptops, iPods, books, clothes and toiletries with you, but they may need to be monitored for contamination before they can be removed from your room. It may sometimes be necessary for us to keep some of your belongings if they are contaminated, but they will be returned to you once they are no longer contaminated.

When can I go home?

The staff from the nuclear medicine or medical physics department will come to the ward to take measurements and they can then work out how much radiation is still in your body and if the level is safe for you to go home. You must stay in your own room until that time. Before going home you may have a whole body scan.

Will I still have any restrictions when I get home?

The nuclear medicine or medical physics staff will explain to you the restrictions you must follow when you go home, for example avoiding crowded places and limiting the people you come into contact with. They can work out exactly how many days you need to restrict yourself. The restrictions you are given may be different from other patients as some patients may be lower or higher in their radioactivity. These restrictions are to protect other people, specially pregnant women and children.

Medical or nursing staff will organise a new supply of thyroid tablets for you to take home and you will be told when to re-start them.

Will I have to come back to the hospital?

You will need to be seen again in the outpatient department by your doctor. You will either be given an appointment when you leave the ward or this may be sent to you later.

When everything is organised, you are free to go home.

Will I need radioactive iodine treatment again?

The treatment may need to be repeated until all the remaining thyroid tissue has been destroyed. Some people require one ablation dose and some people require more than one treatment.

Please remember that this is a low dose of radiation and all these procedures are to protect you and others in case they should need to have radiation treatment in the future. The aim is to keep everybody's radiation exposure to a minimum.

Please contact your specialist treatment centre staff if you have any questions or concerns after reading this information booklet. Together we can help you through your investigations, treatment and recovery.

Useful contacts

The British Thyroid Foundation
PO Box 97, Clifford, Wetherby, West Yorkshire LS23 6XD
Tel: 01423 709707/01423 709448
www.btf-thyroid.org

Butterfly Northeast
PO Box 205, Rowlands Gill, Tyne & Wear NE39 2WX
Tel: 01207 545469
www.butterfly.org.uk

Thyroid Cancer Support UK
www.thyroidcancersupportuk.org

Association for Multiple Endocrine Neoplasia Disorders AMEND (MEN2/FMTC)
31 Pennington Place, Southborough, Kent TN4 0AQ
www.amend.org.uk
email: jo.grey@amend.org.uk

Cancerbackup
Bath Place, Rivington Street, London EC2A 3JR
Tel: 0808 800 1234
www.cancerbackup.org.uk

Macmillan Cancer Support
89 Albert Embankment, London SE1 7UQ
Freephone 0808 808 2020
www.macmillan.org.uk/home.aspx

Cancerlink
Freephone Information Helpline: 0800 132905
www.personal.u-net.com/~njh/cancer.html

CancerHelp UK
www.cancerhelp.org.uk

Thyroid Cancer Survivors' Association
www.thyca.org

Other useful sites can be found in the **British Thyroid Association links page:**
www.btf-thyroid.org